D0453156

BO'NESS

The
Diet
Selector

How to choose a diet perfectly

tailored to your needs

Judith C. Rodriguez

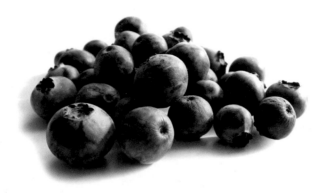

RUNNING PRESS
PHILADELPHIA • LONDON

RUNNING PRESS
PHILADELPHIA • LONDON

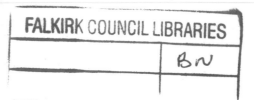
FALKIRK COUNCIL LIBRARIES

Bn

A QUARTO BOOK

Copyright © 2007 Quarto Inc.

Published in 2007 by
Running Press Book Publishers
2300 Chestnut Street
Philadelphia, PA 19103–4371

All rights reserved. No part of this publication may be
reproduced, stored in a retrieval system, or transmitted in
any form or by any means, electronic, mechanical,
photocopying, recording or otherwise, without the prior
permission of the copyright holder.
All product names, company logos, menus, titles and
other distinguishing marks remain the trademark and
copyright of their respective owners.

IBSN-10: 0-7624-3200-4
ISBN-13: 978-0-7624-3200-4

Conceived, designed, and produced by
Quarto Publishing plc
The Old Brewery
6 Blundell Street
London N7 9BH

QUAR.DBI

Project editor: Katie Hallam
Copy editors: Anna Amari-Parker, Bridget Jones
Art director: Caroline Guest
Art editor: Natasha Montgomery
Designer: James Lawrence
Picture research: Claudia Tate

Creative director: Moira Clinch
Publisher: Paul Carslake

Manufactured by PICA Digital
Printed in China by 1010 Printing

10 9 8 7 6 5 4 3 2 1

Visit us on the web! www.runningpresscooks.com

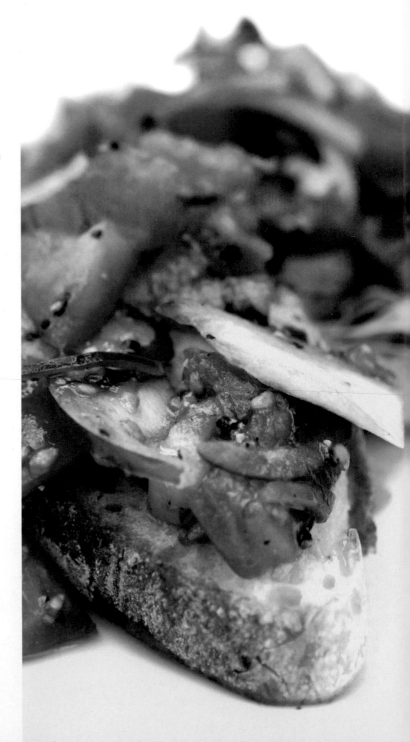

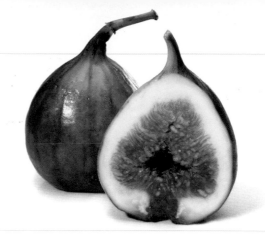

Contents

Diet Directory

WEIGHT-LOSS PLANS 26–129

Behavioural Change

Carb, Protein or Fat Restricted

Commercial and Meal Replacements

Food Focused

Food Groups and Exchanges

Timing or Combination

Other

HEALTH-PROMOTION/ DISEASE-MANAGEMENT PLANS 130–181

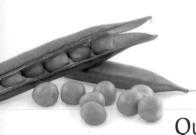

Quick-search alphabetical diet list

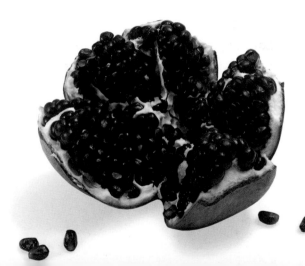

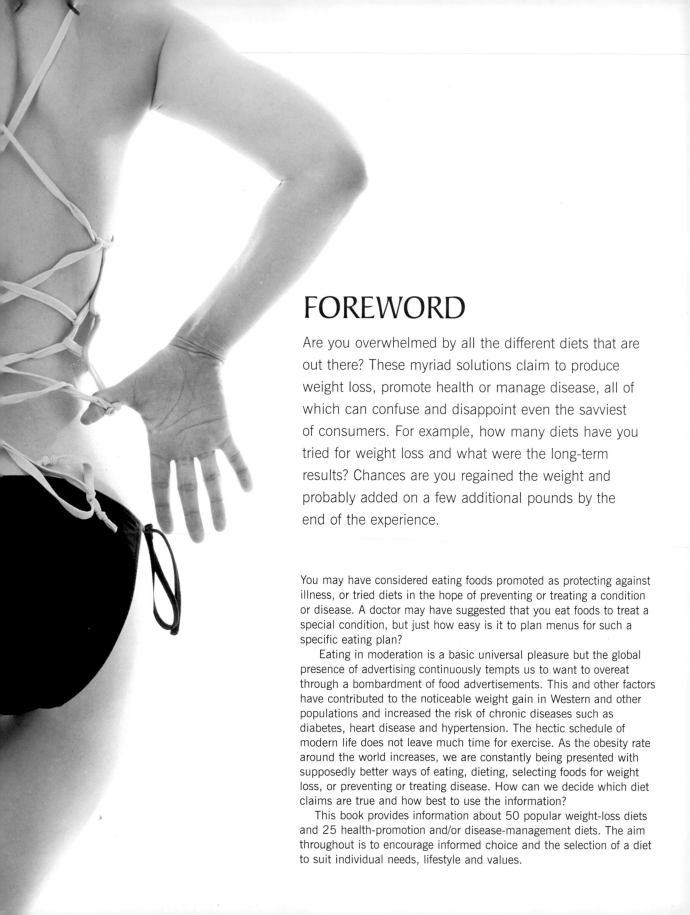

FOREWORD

Are you overwhelmed by all the different diets that are out there? These myriad solutions claim to produce weight loss, promote health or manage disease, all of which can confuse and disappoint even the savviest of consumers. For example, how many diets have you tried for weight loss and what were the long-term results? Chances are you regained the weight and probably added on a few additional pounds by the end of the experience.

You may have considered eating foods promoted as protecting against illness, or tried diets in the hope of preventing or treating a condition or disease. A doctor may have suggested that you eat foods to treat a special condition, but just how easy is it to plan menus for such a specific eating plan?

Eating in moderation is a basic universal pleasure but the global presence of advertising continuously tempts us to want to overeat through a bombardment of food advertisements. This and other factors have contributed to the noticeable weight gain in Western and other populations and increased the risk of chronic diseases such as diabetes, heart disease and hypertension. The hectic schedule of modern life does not leave much time for exercise. As the obesity rate around the world increases, we are constantly being presented with supposedly better ways of eating, dieting, selecting foods for weight loss, or preventing or treating disease. How can we decide which diet claims are true and how best to use the information?

This book provides information about 50 popular weight-loss diets and 25 health-promotion and/or disease-management diets. The aim throughout is to encourage informed choice and the selection of a diet to suit individual needs, lifestyle and values.

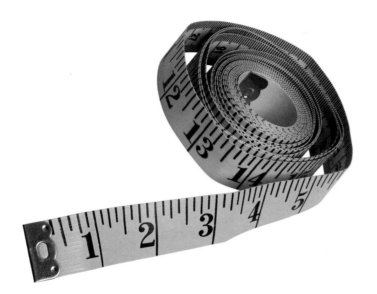

Diet origins and ethos

Diets have been around for a long time and are here to stay. Although it is impossible to determine exactly when or where dieting began, advice has been available for a very long time from a variety of sources and for a range of reasons. Eating limitations and prescriptions originated for different purposes – from fasting for religious rituals to eating to treat illness.

All cultures have ancient teachings on eating for health or on food for treating specific diseases. The Vedas of ancient Hindu scriptures contain teachings that influenced Ayurvedic medicine and modern-day dietary guidelines in Hinduism. Hippocratic theory related health to environmental factors, diet, and living habits, and concepts of ying-yang in Traditional Chinese Medicine (TCM) formed the basis for some popular dietary movements. In recent history, from the sixteenth century to current times, the science of health, diet and nutrition has influenced such concepts. William Harvey-Banting's *Letter on Corpulence* (1864) became the first popular, low-carbohydrate diet to be translated into several languages and sold as a popular diet book.

About the contributors

Simin Bolourchi-Vaghefi, PhD, CNS, is Emeritus Professor of Nutrition of the University of North Florida.

Jenna Braddock, MSH, RD, is a Nutrition Consultant.

Catherine Christie, PhD, RD, is an Associate Professor and Nutrition Program Director at the University of North Florida.

Nancy Correa-Matos, PhD, RD, is an Assistant Professor of Nutrition at the University of North Florida.

Stephanie Perry, MSH, RD, is a Clinical Dietitian and an Adjunct Instructor at the University of North Florida.

Judith C. Rodriguez, PhD, RD, FADA, is Professor of Nutrition at the University of North Florida.

Daniel Santibanez, MPH, RD, is a Clinical Dietitian, Consultant, and Adjunct Instructor at the University of North Florida.

Julia A. Watkins, PhD, RRT, is an Assistant Professor in the Nutrition Program at the University of North Florida.

Sally Weerts, PhD, RD, is an Assistant Professor of Nutrition at the University of North Florida.

Shauna K. Youtz is a graduate of the UNF BSH Nutrition Program.

10 diet myths

1. Skipping meals is a good way to lose weight.

2. Low-fat or zero-fat diets are best for weight loss.

3. The more you cut calories, the better and greater the weight loss.

4. Diet foods are best for weight loss.

5. Starches are fattening.

6. Eating dairy products, bananas and other foods late at night is fattening.

7. Low-fat or fat-free foods are lower in calories.

8. Fast foods cannot be eaten when dieting.

9. Grapefruit, celery and cabbage soup burn fat.

10. Herbal weight-loss products are needed for safe weight loss.

ABOUT THIS BOOK

The chart on page 10 provides an at-a-glance guide to the book's 50 weight-loss diets and 25 health-promotion and disease-management diets. It is ideal for a quick evaluation and overview of the plans most likely to suit your needs. There are five icon ratings to establish each diet's long-term plan or applicability, the effort required, how family friendly it is, the cost involved and how strongly its claims are backed up by the scientific evidence available.

Throughout the sections that follow, there is information about each diet's history, its purported claims and mechanism, the pros and cons that are involved and its relative merits. In addition, resources such as websites, books and a sample menu are included. Regular diet-related "healthy tips" and "weigh this up" boxes help debunk some diet-related myths, and handy "forbidden foods" and "free foods" panels inform you on what you are or are not allowed to eat.

Diet categories

The diets are divided into two major categories: Weight-Loss Plans and Health-Promotion and/or Disease-Management Plans. Although most of the popular diets are for weight loss, despite all their fancy names and claims, most can be classified into one or several categories. For example, a diet may be promoted as "a high-protein plan" but that will probably also make it low in carbohydrates and high in fat. If the diet emphasizes one or more specific foods, it may be included in the food-focused section.

Categories, icons and criteria

LONG-TERM PLAN

● no long-term plan

●● there is an optional, or rudimentary, long-term plan

●●● includes a plan that is adequate for long-term use

FLEXIBILITY

● little or no flexibility for treats and/or food choices

●● optional foods or some flexibility for treats and/or food choices

●●● large number of treats and food choices and/or flexibility which facilitates diet effort

FAMILY FRIENDLY

● the plan is not appropriate for, or should not be used by, other persons

●● some of the restrictions make adoption of the plan difficult

●●● elements of healthy eating that are applicable for, or can be easily modified to suit, family members

A brief history of each diet.

An outline of the claims of the diet and how it works.

An evaluation of possible pros and cons.

Practical aspects of the diet.

At-a-glance ratings system – see below.

An indication of treats and forbidden/free foods.

A handy reference to similar diets.

Useful resources for further information.

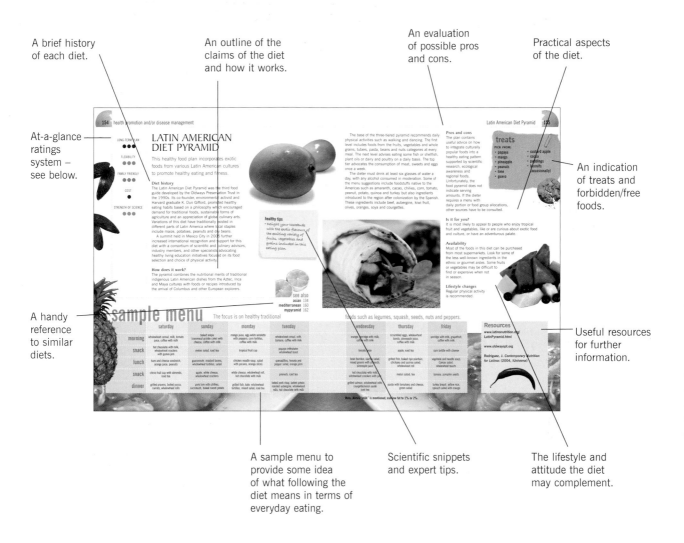

A sample menu to provide some idea of what following the diet means in terms of everyday eating.

Scientific snippets and expert tips.

The lifestyle and attitude the diet may complement.

COST

● can be followed based on the usual cost of foods

●● recommends, or needs, some special items, or includes some fees

●●● needs speciality products (meals, snacks, or supplements) and/or requires fees

STRENGTH OF SCIENCE

● little or no scientific evidence to support the diet's claims or rationale

●● some preliminary, inconclusive, or indirect evidence to support the diet's claims or rationale

●●● strong and/or direct evidence to support the diet's claims or rationale

AT-A-GLANCE EVALUATION GUIDE

KEY

CATEGORIES

Weight-Loss Plans

BC Behavioural Change

R Carbohydrate, Protein or Fat Restricted

C Commercial and Meal Replacements

FF Food Focused

FG Food Groups & Exchanges

TC Timing or Combination

O Other

Health-Promotion/ Disease-Management Plans

HPDM Health Promotion and Disease Management

HP Health Promotion

DM Disease Management

CRITERIA

RATINGS

1 Minimal or least

2 Moderate or some

3 Maximum or most

Weight-Loss Plans	Category	Ratings				
		Adaptability for long-term use	Flexibility for food choices	Adaptability for family members	Level of cost	Level of scientific support
Behavioural Change						
Best Life	BC	3	2	3	2	2
Change One	BC	3	3	3	1	3
French Woman's	BC	3	3	3	1	3
Scentsational	BC	2	3	2	2	1
Supermarket	BC	3	2	3	1	3
Ultimate New York	BC	2	2	1	2	2
You, on a Diet	BC	2	2	2	1	2
Carbohydrate, Protein or Fat Restricted						
Atkins	R	1	3	1	3	2
Complete Hip and Thigh	R	3	2	3	1	2
Dean Ornish	R	2	1	1	1	3
Glycaemic Index	R	3	2	3	1	3
LA Shape	R	2	2	1	2	2
Neanderthin	R	1	1	1	2	1
The New Sugar Busters!	R	2	2	3	1	2
Pritikin	R	2	1	1	1	3
Scarsdale	R	1	1	1	2	1
Secrets of Good-Carb Low-Carb Living	R	3	2	2	1	2
South Beach	R	2	2	2	2	2
Victoria Principal Bikini	R	1	1	1	1	1
Zone	R	1	1	1	2	2
Commercial and Meal Replacements						
Cambridge (excl. Step 1)	C	2	2	2	3	2
Jenny Craig	C	3	2	2	1	3
NutriSystem	C	3	2	2	1	3
OPTIFAST	C	2	1	1	3	2
Slim-Fast	C	1	2	1	2	2
Weight Watchers	C	3	3	3	2	3
Food Focused						
3-Apple-a-Day	FF	2	2	2	1	2
New Cabbage Soup	FF	1	1	1	1	1
Drinking Man's	FF	2	1	1	1	1
Grapefruit	FF	1	2	2	1	1
Juicing	FF	1	1	1	1	1
Peanut Butter	FF	2	3	3	1	3
Food Groups and Exchanges						
Abs	FG	2	2	1	1	2
Bull's-Eye	FG	3	2	3	1	3
Eat, Drink and Weigh Less	FG	2	3	3	1	2
Fat is Not Your Fate	FG	3	3	3	1	3
Mayo	FG	3	3	3	1	3

CATEGORIES

Weight-Loss Plans

BC Behavioural Change

R Carbohydrate, Protein or Fat Restricted

C Commercial and Meal Replacements

FF Food Focused

FG Food Groups & Exchanges

TC Timing or Combination

O Other

Health-Promotion/ Disease-Management Plans

HPDM Health Promotion and Disease Management

HP Health Promotion

DM Disease Management

CRITERIA

RATINGS

1 Minimal or least

2 Moderate or some

3 Maximum or most

Weight-Loss Plans and Health-Promotion/ Disease-Management Plans	Category	Ratings				
		Adaptibility for long-term use	Flexibility for food choices	Adaptibility for family members	Level of cost	Level of scientific support
Food Groups and Exchanges (continued)						
Sonoma	FG	3	3	2	1	2
Tri-Colour	FG	2	3	2	1	3
Volumetrics	FG	3	2	3	1	3
Timing or Combination						
3-Hour	TC	2	2	2	1	2
New Beverly Hills	TC	1	2	1	2	1
Fit for Life	TC	2	2	1	1	1
Grazing	TC	3	3	1	1	2
Hay	TC	1	1	1	1	1
Suzanne Somers	TC	1	2	2	1	1
UltraSimple	TC	1	1	1	2	1
Other						
Eat Right For Your Type	O	2	1	1	1	1
Fasting	O	1	1	1	1	1
Rosedale	O	2	2	1	3	2
Health-Promotion/Disease-Management Plans						
Additive-Free	HPDM	2	1	2	2	2
Asian Diet Pyramid	HP	3	2	3	2	3
Candida	HPDM	1	1	1	1	1
DASH	HPDM	3	3	3	1	3
Elimination	DM	3	1	1	2	3
GERD	DM	3	3	3	1	3
Gluten-Free	DM	3	2	2	1	3
Good Mood	HP	3	2	3	1	3
Intuitive Eating	HP	3	3	3	1	3
Lacto-Ovo Vegetarian	HP	3	3	3	1	3
Lactose-Restricted	DM	3	2	3	1	3
Latin American	HP	3	3	3	1	3
Low-Sodium	HPDM	3	2	3	1	3
Master Cleanser	HP	1	1	1	1	1
Mediterranean	HP	3	3	3	1	3
MyPyramid	HP	3	3	3	1	3
Omega Plan	HP	3	2	3	1	2
Overeaters Anonymous	DM	3	3	3	1	3
Perricone Promise	HP	2	2	1	2	2
Pregnancy	HP	3	3	3	1	3
Rainbow	HP	3	3	3	1	3
Raw Food	HP	2	1	1	2	1
TLC	HPDM	3	3	3	1	3
Vegan	HP	3	3	2	2	3
What Would Jesus Eat?	HP	3	2	3	1	3

DIETING TODAY

According to the World Health Organization (WHO), worldwide more than one billion adults are overweight and at least three hundred million of them are obese. In the US about 64 per cent of the population are overweight, and Europe (traditionally considered to have a leaner population) is catching up fast. It is expected that the US overweight population will be at about 70 per cent in 2009. In Europe this figure will have grown from about 48 per cent to over 50 per cent by 2009.

Overall, people are eating more food than ever before and leading less strenuous lives physically. Modern-day convenience appliances may be helping us to save energy in the environment but they do not encourage us to use up the calories (energy) in our bodies. All these factors are contributing to the growing rate of overweight and obese individuals around the world.

Supersize me

20 years ago	today
Bagel was 7.5cm across and 140 calories	Bagel is 5cm across and 350 calories
Turkey sandwich was 320 calories	Turkey sandwich has 820 calories
Fizzy drink was 185ml and 85 calories	Fizzy drink is about 570ml and 250 calories
Serving of French fries was 70g and 210 calories	Serving of French fries is 200g and 610 calories
Chicken Caesar salad was 150g and 390 calories	Chicken Caesar salad is about 300g and 790 calories

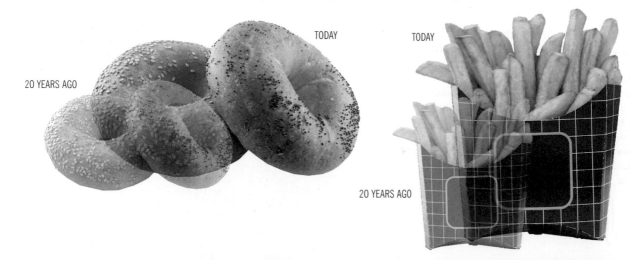

TODAY

TODAY

20 YEARS AGO

20 YEARS AGO

Diet figures

It is estimated that at any point in time about 40 per cent of women and 20 per cent of men are on a diet. Over a lifetime, dieting behaviour occurs in about 50 per cent of men and 75 per cent of women. Although women are more likely to have tried a variety of diets, the prevalence of both overweight and dieting individuals is increasing across both genders. Slightly more than 30 per cent of dieters use supplements as a part of their weight-loss efforts. Regardless of how weight reduction is promoted, the levels of satisfaction with these diets are low. One study found that only 17 per cent of respondents were pleased with the diets they had tried.

Dieting is not only for weight loss but also for improved health. About 70 per cent of dieters aim to improve their health. One US study – the Continuing Survey of Food Intakes by Individuals (CSFII 1994–96) – found that about 71 per cent of dieters are dieting to improve health and about 50 per cent to lose weight.

More books: more weight

No wonder weight-loss and diet books are popular. Ironically, the popularity of diet books has accompanied weight increase, not reduction. In general, Americans currently spend more on weight control products than Europeans (£75 versus £60 per head in 2004). However, it is expected that European growth will outstrip the US over the next five years. Finding ways to halt it is a growing international concern. As obesity continues to increase and dieting becomes a global preoccupation in the developed world, the prevalence of eating disorders has also grown.

Obesity and chronic disease

Lifestyle changes and an increase in the number of people who are overweight have also contributed to the rise of the many chronic diseases for which special diets are necessary. Being obese and overweight are risk factors for cardiovascular disease, type 2 diabetes and certain types of cancer. Obesity and being overweight may also aggravate other conditions such as gall bladder disease, respiratory problems, osteoarthritis and hypertension.

Fad diet timeline

1820	Vinegar and Water Diet	Made popular by Lord Byron
1825	Low-Carbohydrate Diet	First appeared in the *Physiology of Taste* by Jean Brillat-Savarin
1830	Graham's Diet	Only legacy: invented Graham cracker
1863	Banting's Low-Carbohydrate Diet	"Banting" became a popular term for dieting
1903	Horace Fletcher promotes "Fletcherizing"	Chew food 32 times
1917	Calorie Counting	Introduced by Lulu Hunt Peters in her book *Diet and Health, with Key to the Calories*
1925	Cigarette Diet	"Reach for a Lucky instead of a sweet"
1928	Inuit Meat and Fat Diet	Caribou, raw fish and whale blubber
1930	Hay Diet	Carbohydrates and proteins not allowed during the same meal
	Dr Stoll's Diet Aid	First of the liquid diet drinks
1934	Bananas and Skimmed Milk Diet	Backed by the United Fruit Company
1950	Cabbage Soup Diet	Flatulence listed as a main side effect
	Grapefruit Diet	Also known as the Hollywood Diet
1960	Zen Macrobiotic Diet	Created by Japanese philosopher George Ohsawa
1961	Calories Don't Count Diet	US Food and Drug Administration filed charges regarding the diet's claims
1964	Drinking Man's Diet	Harvard School of Public Health declared the diet unhealthy
1970	Sleeping Beauty Diet	Individuals heavily sedated for several days
	Liquid Protein Diets	Liquid protein drinks were low in vitamins and minerals
1981	Beverly Hills Diet	Only fruit for 10 days but in unlimited amounts
1985	Fit for Life	Avoid combining protein and carbohydrate foods
	Caveman Diet	Foods from the Paleolithic Era
1986	Rotation Diet	Rotating number of calories taken in from week to week
1987	Scarsdale Diet	Low-carbohydrate, low-calorie diet plan
1990	Cabbage Soup Diet	Diet from the 1950s resurfaces on the Internet
1994	High-Protein, Low-Carb Diet	Dr Atkin's version
1995	Sugar Busters – Cut Sugar to Trim Fat	Eliminates refined carbohydrates
1996	Eat Right For Your Type	Diet based on blood type
1999	Juice, Fasting and Detoxification	Perennial dieting favorites reappear in combination
2000	Raw Food Diet	Focuses on uncooked, unprocessed organic foods
2001	High-Protein, Low-Carb Diet	1994 diet updated
2004	Coconut Diet	Fats replaced with coconut oil
2005	Cheater's Diet	Cheating on the weekend is required
2006	Maple Syrup Diet	Features a special lemon syrup drink

Fad Diet Timeline. Copyright 2007 American Dietetic Association. Reprinted with permission.

MAKING THE MOST OF YOUR DIET

The Diet Selector will even help you evaluate diets beyond the scope of this book. By applying the information given, other diets can be categorized and assessed for their rationale, pros and cons, strength of the science and suitability. When evaluating any diet, it is ultimately important to consider nutritional adequacy, variety, moderation, proportionality (appropriate amounts from different food groups), gradual improvement, application to lifestyle, suitability for long-term use (or over your lifetime) and the inclusion of physical activity.

Promoting health

The best strategy for encouraging health and maintaining a healthy weight is to choose a lifestyle that you can live with for the rest of your life and that is conducive to good health. A healthy lifestyle will need to include daily physical activity that you enjoy such as walking, cycling or dancing, and can also include day-to-day chores such as gardening or mopping. It must also include eating a variety of minimally processed foods in moderation so as to eat the required nutrients. In an effort to guide populations towards healthy food choices, many food options have been developed.

As we try to take care of our health and seek to prevent illness and disease, we may try various diets that are now classified as disease preventing or health promoting plans. For countries in which chronic diseases, such as heart disease, stroke, cancer, diabetes, chronic respiratory diseases and hypertension, are among the major causes of death, there has been an increased move towards health promotion and disease prevention by managing risk factors, which often includes diet, as well as avoiding excessive alcohol intake and smoking.

Managing disease

A diet component is included in the management of many common diseases or illnesses. This can help delay the progression of the condition which is important for quality of life. The following diets, often prescribed for disease management, are discussed in the book: additive-free,

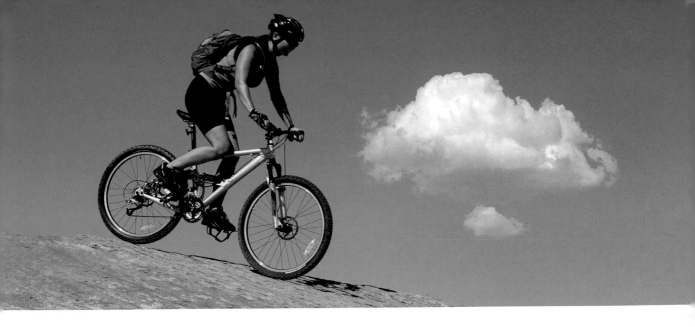

allergy or elimination, dietary approaches to hypertension (DASH), gastro-oesophageal reflux disease (GERD), gluten-free, low sodium and therapeutic lifestyle change (TLC). Several other popular diets used by consumers for a variety of reasons are discussed as well as the evidence for their rationale.

These chronic conditions pose tremendous costs to both the individual and society. The global cost of chronic diseases (which have superseded communicable diseases as the leading cause of death in the developed world) pose an enormous financial burden on both the individual and society because around 80 per cent of the world's population live in areas where chronic diseases are now the major cause of death. As a result, the emphasis is on the prevention of disease and the promotion of health. From a policy perspective, health promotion involves providing consumers with eating and lifestyle behaviour guidelines that can be easily understood and followed. The adoption of healthy behaviours, such as eating food appropriate to an illness, participating in appropriate physical activity, and, if required, taking the necessary medications, will minimize the progression of disease.

Losing weight
Most of the weight-loss diets reviewed in this book provide temporary weight loss because, regardless of the plan or claim, they are basically low in calories. Here lies the limitation, since this temporary loss will be primarily water for many of the diets. The scientific evidence consistently concludes that successful weight loss should include a plan that enables the dieter to manage weight over his or her lifetime. The more extreme the plan, the more difficult it is to stay on track for the long term. The key for lifelong success is following a plan that is tailored to meet your needs. Research indicates that calorie- and portion-restricted diets may have easier "sticking power" than fat- and carbohydrate-restricted diets.

Weight loss ultimately occurs because there is caloric restriction and compliance to the diet. For weight loss that stays off over the long term, the calorie restriction cannot come into conflict with preferred foods, and the plan must have a transitional phase that allows for a shift to a healthy plan that can be followed for life. An active lifestyle will also help maintain a reasonable weight and provide physical fitness.

Maintaining a healthy weight
Generally people put themselves on a diet for a short time rather than permanently change their eating habits. They then come off the diet after losing weight and revert back to the behaviour patterns that caused the weight to pile on in the first place. The solution to losing weight and keeping it off long term is a factor with two components: the energy or amount of calories consumed as food and the energy expended in physical activity. Eating more calories than those used will result in weight gain, while using more calories than those eaten will lead to weight loss. Keeping this basic principle in mind, the idea is to match your weight-loss programme and activity to your daily schedule, provided it is safe and effective.

The objective of losing weight should really be to reduce the percentage of body fat. Although most weight-loss efforts are aimed at gaining a more attractive figure, it is important to realize that the ultimate goal is to preserve health and prevent the damage caused by an excess of body fat. Any weight-loss plan should aim to reduce this excess body fat which is a risk factor for heart disease, hypertension, type 2 diabetes and some types of cancer.

HOW TO LOSE WEIGHT

The sad truth is that most of us are overweight or obese because we eat too much and are far too sedentary. While genetics, a slower metabolic rate and other factors may play a role, it is generally a small one. The following are possible factors:

- An increase in the consumption of high-calorie (energy-dense) foods, especially those purchased and eaten away from home.
- Certain behavioural patterns such as a rigid restraint followed by periodic overeating.
- The excessive consumption of processed foods with high levels of refined sugars and fats.
- A surplus of sedentary activities, such as watching television, or working and playing at the computer.
- Larger portion sizes.
- A low consumption of high-fibre foods such as fruits, vegetables and wholegrain foods.

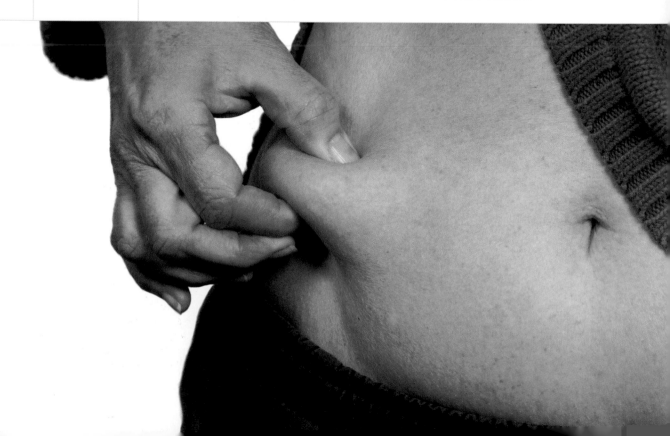

Weight and metabolism

The thyroid helps to regulate metabolism. When this gland is overactive (hyperthyroidism), metabolism increases and causes weight loss. If the thyroid gland is underactive (hypothyroidism), metabolism slows down with weight gain as a side effect. But although thyroid activity is related to metabolism, in reality a very small amount of weight gain is attributable to hypothyroidism.

A healthy weight range

Although there are various quick ways to determine if weight is likely to increase the risk of disease, all methods for risk determination mean different things and must be evaluated accordingly.

Body mass index (BMI) This number is determined using a formula that incorporates height and weight. It is a good estimate but is not a useful measure for those who are very muscular. A BMI of 19–24.9 is considered healthy, 25–29.9 is overweight and 30 and above is considered obese.

Waist-to-hip ratio This measure helps determine the body's fat pattern and distribution. To determine this ratio, measure the waist and hip circumference. Divide the waist value by the hip value. If the waist-to-hip ratio is greater than 0.90 for a male or 0.80 for a female, the person is considered to be at higher risk of some diseases.

Waist size This measure helps indicate how the body fat is distributed (distribution is associated with risk for some conditions). A waist size over 89 centimetres (35 inches) for women and 100 centimetres (40 inches) for men indicates an overweight individual.

Other checks There are other ways to determine body fat levels, for example weight scales or other instruments are available to calculate body fat by using a method called bioelectrical impedance. Another technique, which requires a skilled individual, is the skin-fold thickness test. A more costly, less available method involves underwater weighing.

A healthy weight for women would include a body fat range of 15 to 25 per cent and 10 to 20 per cent for men. Over 25 per cent body fat for women and over 20 per cent body fat for men are regarded as indicators of overweight.

Approaches to weight loss

How effective are most dietary strategies for weight loss in the long term? The research is not conclusive but seems to indicate that most weight loss diets are ineffective unless they include changes in physical activity as well as food habits. There are many popular diets that provide a   >

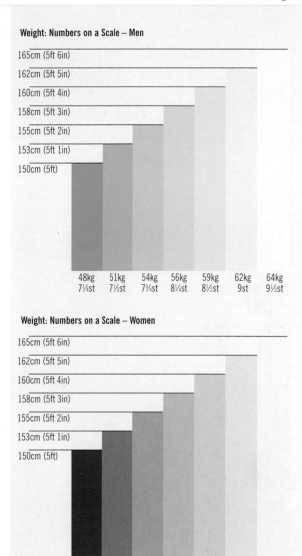

Weight These charts do not indicate levels of fitness. However, increased weight has been associated with an increased risk for some conditions, so weight charts can give a quick estimate of possible fitness level. For men, calculate 106 pounds for the first 5 feet, plus 6 pounds for every inch over 5 feet (or minus 6 pounds for every inch below 5 feet). For women, calculate 100 pounds for 5 feet and 5 additional pounds for every inch over 5 feet (or minus 5 pounds for every inch below 5 feet). You should subtract or add 10 per cent to that number to get the high and low weight ranges.

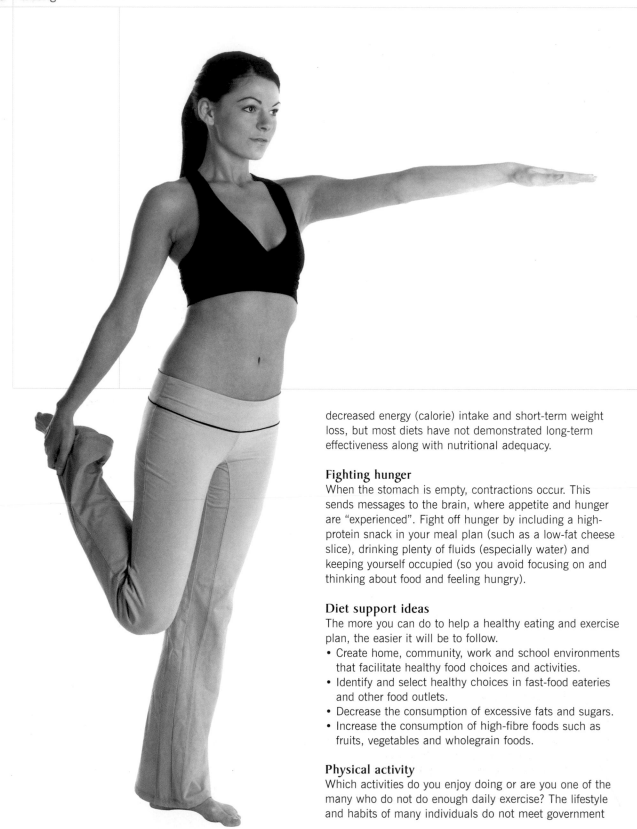

decreased energy (calorie) intake and short-term weight loss, but most diets have not demonstrated long-term effectiveness along with nutritional adequacy.

Fighting hunger

When the stomach is empty, contractions occur. This sends messages to the brain, where appetite and hunger are "experienced". Fight off hunger by including a high-protein snack in your meal plan (such as a low-fat cheese slice), drinking plenty of fluids (especially water) and keeping yourself occupied (so you avoid focusing on and thinking about food and feeling hungry).

Diet support ideas

The more you can do to help a healthy eating and exercise plan, the easier it will be to follow.
- Create home, community, work and school environments that facilitate healthy food choices and activities.
- Identify and select healthy choices in fast-food eateries and other food outlets.
- Decrease the consumption of excessive fats and sugars.
- Increase the consumption of high-fibre foods such as fruits, vegetables and wholegrain foods.

Physical activity

Which activities do you enjoy doing or are you one of the many who do not do enough daily exercise? The lifestyle and habits of many individuals do not meet government

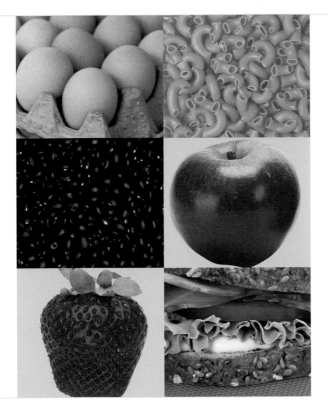

recommendations. For example, although Britons seem to be eating more healthily, less than half of them meet the recommended 150 minutes of weekly activity levels. In the US the general recommendation is about 30 minutes of exercise a day but it is estimated that only about 46 per cent meet the recommendation and 24 per cent are physically inactive.

Many of us have been seduced into believing that being active means owning exercise equipment, joining a gym or participating in strenuous workouts. Physical activity can be easily incorporated into daily life such as brief walks throughout the day, dancing or even routines such as walking on the spot whilst listening to the radio or watching television. The key is to enjoy the activity as part of your daily routine. This will prevent it from feeling like a burden, chore or punishment.

Other weight-loss methods

Although diet and exercise are the usual and preferred methods for treating obesity, prescription medications and/or surgery may be recommended for morbidly obese persons in extreme cases. Medications such as Sibutramine (Reductil) and Orlistat (Xenical) might be prescribed to assist with weight loss. They should only be taken under medical supervision since they have potential side effects. Some have been withdrawn from the market, for example fenfluramine and dexfenfluramine, because of their potential life-threatening effects.   >

10 ways to increase daily activity

1. Do stretching exercises to increase flexibility before, during or after taking a shower.

2. Use the toilet that is further away.

3. Do alternate leg extensions and bring your feet almost level with your knees when sitting (while watching television, for example).

4. Pace or walk on the spot whilst talking on the telephone.

5. Park further away and walk or jog to the door.

6. Take the stairs whenever you have less than three flights to walk.

7. Do star jumps while waiting for your food to cook.

8. Go and talk to a colleague instead of sending an email.

9. Sweep, mop and/or garden daily, or play a game with your children.

10. Dance to two or three songs in the morning or evening.

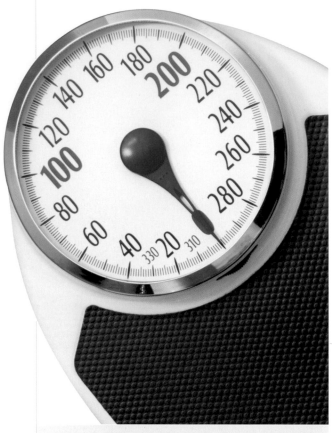

5 steps to creating your own diet

1. Identify a measure and decide on a goal based on it, for example BMI, body fat or weight.

2. Identify and implement daily ways to eat less and exercise more.

3. Plan when you eat and what you eat: breakfast like a king, lunch like a prince and dinner like a pauper.

4. Determine how much you should eat: portion control and plate size.

5. Determine ways to include your favourite treats.

Surgical procedures are limited to the morbidly obese and may include vertical banded gastroplasty, gastric bypass or gastric banding. Gastroplasty involves stapling a small section of the stomach. During a gastric bypass intervention, the lower part of the small intestine is stapled to the stomach so less food is absorbed due to it bypassing the stomach. In gastric banding the size of the stomach is reduced by using a constricting band.

Disordered eating

There is a variety of chaotic eating patterns with a range of potential health complications. Yo-yo dieting is a term for a pattern of gaining and losing weight that results from constant dieting. This is taxing on the body and, depending on overall health, may be hazardous.

In some cases, food can take on extreme significance and this may result in anorexia, a form of extreme self-starvation that results from a distorted body image. In spite of being extremely thin, the sufferer will see herself or himself as overweight and will engage obsessively in exercise and starvation to lose an alarming amount of weight, thereby becoming seriously ill, and in some cases can even die. Bulimia nervosa involves (usually secret) cycles of bingeing and purging. Laxatives, enemas, excessive exercise or other harmful behaviours may be used to obtain relief from the guilt associated with bingeing. Binge eating disorder is similar to bulimia nervosa but does not include purging.

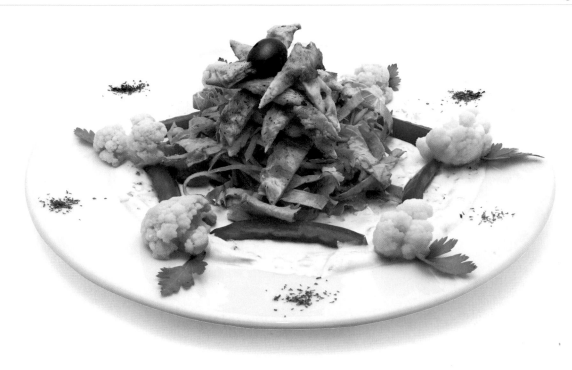

Although disordered eating is more common among women, it is also prevalent in men and increasing in prevalence overall. If you suspect someone has disordered eating, advise the person to seek professional help.

Successful long-term weight management

The term "diet" evokes thoughts of something temporary. This "on-and-off" behaviour only produces transitional change and does not address the underlying behaviours that created the need to diet in the first place. The best programmes for weight reduction and health promotion that help to reduce body weight and fat with lasting results are the ones that accomplish the following objectives: gradually but consistently decreasing energy (calorie) intake from foods and increasing energy (calorie) expenditure through physical activity. It is important to remember that physical exercise builds up muscles and plays a key role in utilizing body fat reserves for energy.

Diets that promise immediate or fast results are not to be trusted as they defy the scientific basis for the body's metabolism. Such claims are misleading and potentially harmful. A simple calculation of energy balance will establish that you cannot safely lose more than half to one kilogram (one to two pounds) per week, even if you starve yourself. For example, to lose half a kilogram (one pound) of body fat you will need to have a "negative or calorie deficit of 3,500 calories", a daily caloric reduction (by decreasing intake or increasing physical activity) of   >

No secrets: 5 steps for lifelong health promotion

1. **Identify and implement some simple, positive diet and physical activity changes that you can commit to.**

2. **Don't smoke.**

3. **Drink alcohol only in moderation.**

4. **Maintain a healthy body weight.**

5. **Get regular medical check-ups and health screenings, especially if you are at risk of heart disease, cancer, diabetes, hypertension or osteoporosis.**

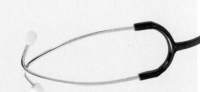

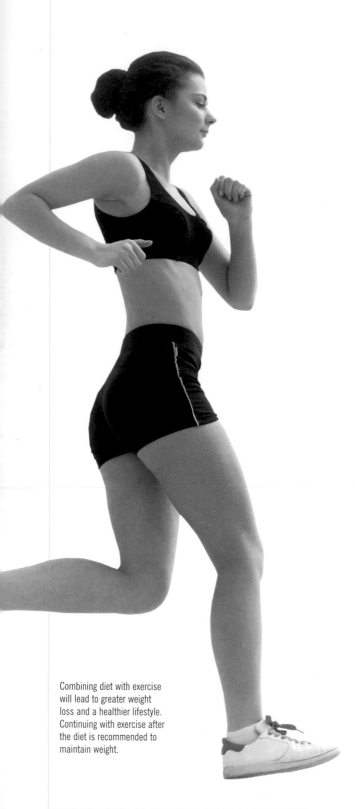

Combining diet with exercise will lead to greater weight loss and a healthier lifestyle. Continuing with exercise after the diet is recommended to maintain weight.

500 calories per day. So, if your usual daily calorie intake is 2,000 calories, you need to reduce your intake by 500 calories per day to lose half a kilo in a week. Even if you starve yourself by drinking water without eating, you will only lose two kilograms (four pounds) a week. But that is neither safe nor wise. Your body will lose muscle and water, important body components, putting itself at risk.

Dieting must have a serious objective and should not be casually undertaken. Before going on a restrictive eating plan, obtain the approval of your GP or other healthcare provider and have a health check-up to make sure it is safe to proceed. When the habitual food intake is changed, some metabolic changes start to occur in the body after just a couple of weeks of being on a low-calorie or restricted-calorie diet. A reduction in caloric intake acts as a signal for the metabolic rate to go down as the body starts adapting to having reduced energy available for physiological function and economizes on calorie expenditure to compensate. In weight-loss diets, this is called a weight plateau. To overcome this situation, an increase in physical activity or an even greater reduction in calorie intake is suggested. The best way to get over the plateau is to increase physical activity and reduce calorie intake simultaneously.

When planning a diet, choose one that can be adapted to your lifestyle and health needs. It should work for a long time. Remember that going on and off a diet and regressing back to your old eating habits will result in the weight lost being regained or could negatively impact on the progression of a disease.

Health promotion and disease management

Health promotion is the attempt at controlling and improving health by managing factors related to lifestyle such as diet, physical activity, stress and environment to maximize quality of life.

Chronic worldwide diseases such as heart disease, stroke, cancer, respiratory diseases and diabetes are the leading causes of death and disability in the west. Most are impacted by or have their progression and severity minimized by diet; many can be avoided by healthy eating habits. One major diet-related culprit is the increased consumption of energy-dense (high-calorie) foods that are high in sugar, and/or saturated fats and/or salt. These foods are associated with an increased risk of developing many chronic diseases. Factors such as high cholesterol, high blood pressure, obesity and alcohol dependency can be changed through dietary habits and physical activity. The scientific research indicates that appropriate and sustained behavioural intervention can reduce the risk of chronic disease.

No secrets: 5 steps to lifelong weight management

1 Eat food in the appropriate portion sizes.
• Meat, poultry and fish servings about the size of a pack of cards or bar of soap.
• Pasta, rice and other grains about the size of a tennis ball (half if trying to cut calories).
• Vegetables about the size of a tennis ball; legumes about half of a tennis ball.
• A piece of cheese equal to about four dice.

2 Focus on slow, gradual weight loss through regular eating and physical activity.

3 Eat a variety of foods with an emphasis on lots of different whole grains, fruits, vegetables, low-fat dairy products, lean poultry, meats, fish, legumes, nuts and seeds.

4 Drink plenty of water.

5 Limit fats, added sugars and refined foods.

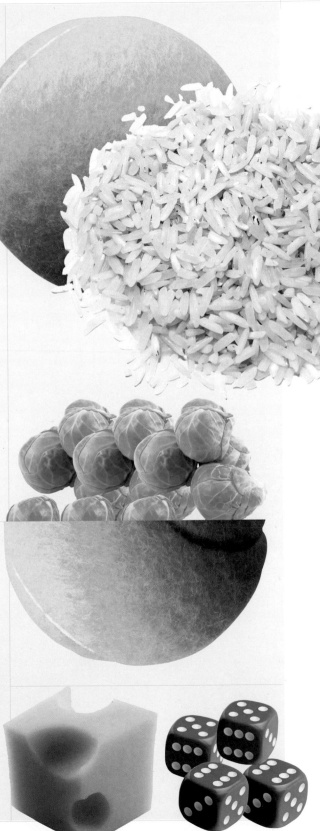

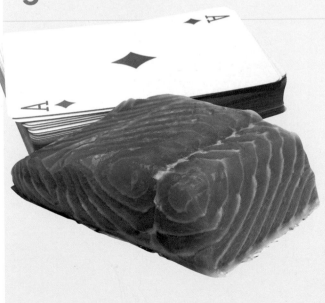

ESSENTIAL NOTES

Quick-reference calorie counter

230g thick vanilla shake = 256 calories
245g skimmed milk = 83 calories
230g low-fat fruit yogurt = 225 calories
230g plain skimmed milk yogurt = 127 calories
105g rich vanilla ice cream = 266 calories
75g low-fat vanilla ice cream = 125 calories

2 pieces (163g) commercial breaded fried chicken wings = 494 calories
80g grilled sirloin steak = 218 calories
80g grilled sirloin cut lamb chop = 200 calories
80g roast pork tenderloin steak =139 calories
80g grilled tuna = 118 calories
80g steamed prawns = 84 calories

1 can (340ml) standard cola = 136 calories
1 can (340ml) standard iced tea = 128 calories
230ml unsweetened grapefruit juice = 94 calories
230ml fruit-flavoured sports drink = 66 calories
1 can (340ml) low-calorie cola = 4 calories
1 bottle water = 0 calories

1 small serving chips (74g) = 245 calories
1 medium sweet potato, baked (114g) = 103 calories
1 large orange (184g) = 86 calories
1 medium apple (138g) with skin = 72 calories
90g cooked spinach = 21 calories
62g cooked cauliflower = 14 calories

1 slice (125g) commercial apple pie = 296 calories
1 piece (64g) chocolate cake with icing = 235 calories
1 medium glazed doughnut (45g) = 192 calories
3 sponge fingers (33g) = 120 calories
1 piece angel cake (28g) = 72 calories
2 low-fat vanilla waters (12g) = 53 calories

55g dry roasted peanuts = 332 calories
55g crisps = 310 calories
55g roasted soya beans = 271 calories
55g pretzel sticks = 215 calories
2 brown rice cakes (18g) = 70 calories
122g carrot sticks = 50 calories

USDA Nutrient Data Laboratory

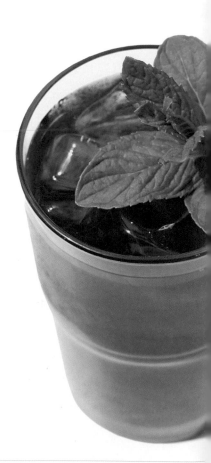

Metric/imperial conversions

to convert	to	divide by
grams	ounces	28.3495
kilograms	pounds	0.4536
litres	pint (dry)	0.5506
litres	pint (liquid)	0.4732
litres	quart (dry)	1.1012
litres	quart (liquid)	0.9463
litres	gallons	3.7853
centimetres	inches	2.54
metres	feet	0.3048

Tips for breaking the exercise barrier

5 reasons why you don't exercise	What to do about it
1. You're too busy.	Put exercise into your schedule and give it priority. Exercise while you watch TV and incorporate activities into daily routines, like using the stairs at work.
2. You don't like it.	Identify things you like to do and use those for exercise, such as dancing and walking with friends.
3. You feel too fat to move.	Start slowly with some chair-based exercises, yoga and some mild stretching.
4. It's too tiring.	Don't do too much at the beginning. Try doing 10 minutes 2–3 times a day.
5. You don't have money for equipment or memberships.	You don't need to buy special equipment or join fancy clubs. Use food tins or jugs filled with water as weights, and use a rope for skipping.

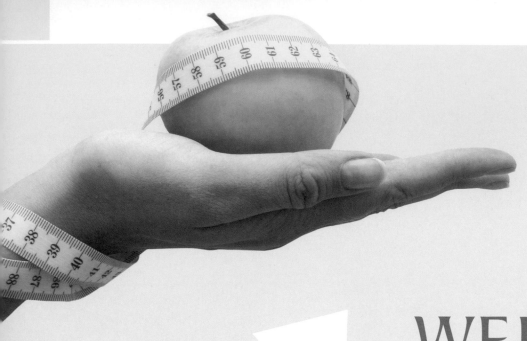

WEIGHT-

The weight-loss plans in this book are categorized into the following seven major types:

- **Behavioural** plans focus on a variety of strategies that might include diet, physical activity and/or stress management.
- **Food-focused** plans emphasize eating one or several foods.
- **Low-carbohydrate, low-protein or low-fat** plans are grouped together since their focus is on limiting one or more of the macronutrients (carbohydrates, proteins and fats).
- **Food groups, guides or exchange systems** are emphasized in some eating programmes.
- **The timing or combination** of meals and snacks are the focus of certain diet plans.
- **Commercial meal or snack replacements** are used in some dieting methods.
- **Other** diets include unique plans.

The categories are based on some common principles (such as sharing the low-carbohydrate characteristic), even though authors may use different classifications. For example, the Somers Diet was classified under "timing or combination" but it has also been referred to as a "celebrity diet".

LOSS PLANS

Fascinating facts

There are many types of weight-loss diet, including the following:

- Behavioural change or behaviour modification plans
- Blood type diets
- Celebrity diets
- Clinically supervised diets
- Commercial plans
- Exchange plans
- Fad diets
- Fasting or juicing diets
- Genetic type diets
- Food group or food guide plans
- Food-focused or food-specific diets
- High-fibre or volumetric diets
- High-protein diets

- Lifestyle diets
- Low-calorie diets
- Low-carbohydrate diets
- Low-fat diets
- Low-glycaemic index diets
- Low-protein diets
- Meal-replacement plans
- Restriction diets
- Time or meal-combination diets

Many diets can be a combination of these. For example, a low-fat diet may also be low-carbohydrate, so it actually becomes a high-protein diet, and a low-glycaemic index diet may also include food exchanges.

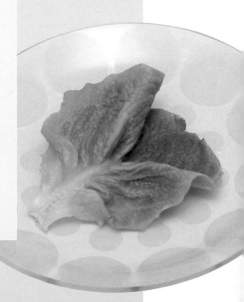

It is important to drink at least eight glasses of water per day.

LONG-TERM PLAN

FLEXIBILITY

FAMILY FRIENDLY

COST

STRENGTH OF SCIENCE

BEST LIFE DIET

A three-phase plan to definitive weight loss through behavioural changes, increased activity levels, improvements in diet and the resolution of key eating issues.

Diet history

Although Bob Greene, an exercise physiologist, published this diet programme in 2006, it only really became popular after being featured on *The Oprah Winfrey Show*. The Best Life plan's practical approach stands to gain even more widespread popularity due to its celebrity following.

How does it work?

This three-phase programme gradually eases the person dieting into a healthier diet and a more active lifestyle.

Phase 1 lasts a minimum of four weeks and focuses on increasing the individual's metabolism by adding and increasing the frequency of exercise. This stage includes three structured mealtimes and not consuming food within two hours of going to sleep.

The focus of Phase 2, which should last a minimum of four weeks, involves weight loss, cutting calories and changing food choices. In reality, significant weight loss is not expected to occur until Phase 2 due to increasing levels of exercise, the removal of nutrient-poor,

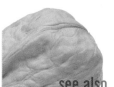

see also
south beach 64
mediterranean 160
tlc 176

sample menu

When shopping, look for the Best Life seal.

	saturday	sunday	monday	tuesday
morning	spinach and red or green pepper omelette, 100g fresh berries, low-fat yogurt	traditional porridge with chopped dried fruit and nuts, 240ml skimmed milk	mocha coffee with skimmed milk, 1 high-fibre muffin, 1 apple	Kashi® cereal with nuts, 240ml skimmed milk, ½ grapefruit
lunch	tabbouleh with lean meat chunks	wholewheat pitta stuffed with lean turkey and vegetables, 1 citrus fruit	veggie and bean wrap on a wholewheat tortilla, green salad with vinaigrette dressing	peanut butter and pear sandwich with wholegrain bread, 75g carrots
supper	vegetable soup, Mediterranean-style prawns with tomatoes, 1 citrus fruit	beef or chicken fajitas, seasoned steamed vegetable	wholewheat pasta with marinara sauce, grilled chicken, green salad with vinaigrette dressing	lemon-grilled fish, small ear of corn, sugar snap peas
snack 1	banana-coffee smoothie	high-fibre cereal and 240ml skimmed or soya milk	wholegrain crackers and low-fat cheese	170ml yogurt with sprinkled nuts
snack 2	small bowl of fruit sorbet	low-fat ice cream with drizzle of chocolate sauce	small piece of dark chocolate	low-fat ice cream

unhealthy foods, becoming attuned to the cues that provoke the hunger signal and assessing the emotional reasons for overeating.

Phase 3 is centred on finding lifelong fitness levels to suit the individual and fine-tuning his or her corresponding diet. This final stage is designed to last for "the rest of your life".

Permanent weight maintenance and stabilization is encouraged through improved food choices and achieving a good understanding of their nutritional value. The "Anything Goes Calories" concept is introduced to fit in favourite kinds of food too so the selection is not so overly restrictive. The scientific evidence supports the effectiveness of weight-loss plans that combine diet and physical activity, and behavioural strategies or permanent healthy diet and weight management.

Pros and cons

The Best Life Diet focuses on sustained weight loss by underlining the importance of assessing the emotional reasons for overeating. Although the plan deals with emotional eating issues on a self-help basis, it may be advisable to seek professional counselling on specific eating issues.

The book refers the reader to its affiliated website, which offers a pay-as-you-go subscription service for a monthly fee. A 10-day risk-free trial is also available. Although some information is available for free, access to the vast majority of the tips and recipes requires subscription privileges.

Is it for you?

This diet is suitable for individuals who are seeking to develop a permanently healthier lifestyle in their quest to lose and keep the weight off without resorting to faddy gimmicks. It might not appeal to anyone seeking a fast method of weight loss who does not want to (or cannot) participate in physical activity.

Availability

Most foods in this diet are available from your local grocery store or supermarket. The programme and several well-known food companies – Green Giant®, Yoplait®, Cascadian Farms®, and Cheerios® to name just a few – have teamed up to produce the instantly recognizable Best Life seal of approval on diet-approved products.

Lifestyle changes

Behaviour modification and physical activity constitute the foundation of this life plan.

healthy tips
• The only food group that is encouraged liberally on this plan is vegetables without any added fats.

wednesday	thursday	friday	Resources
fruit and soya milk smoothie, 1 slice wholegrain bread with peanut butter	low-fat yogurt topped with high-fibre cereal, walnuts and fresh fruit	high-fibre cereal bar, skimmed or soya milk, piece of fruit, 3 tbsp nuts	www.thebestlife.com
green salad with chicken and fresh fruit, wholewheat crackers and low-fat cheese	Greek-style wholewheat pitta sandwich, 75g carrots, ½ serving of citrus fruit	grilled chicken, bean and spinach salad with low-calorie dressing, 1 wholegrain roll	www.eatbetteramerica.com
green salad, steak and cheese crumbles, baked sweet potato, low-fat plain yogurt and sour cream	Southwest chicken salad, small serving baked tortilla chips	Oriental chicken and vegetable stir-fry, brown rice	**Green, B. The Best Life Diet (2006, Simon & Schuster)**
handful of almonds, latte coffee drink with skimmed milk	high-protein, low-calorie chocolate shake	wholegrain crackers with fruit jam, 240ml skimmed milk	
light popcorn	35g chocolate-covered nuts	1 serving baked vegetable chips	

CHANGE ONE DIET

As its name implies, this weight-loss plan emphasizes adjusting one factor at a time, plus advocates portion control and managing aspects of daily life that are related to food choices.

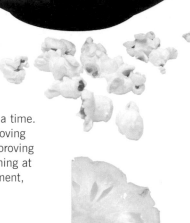

Diet history
The plan was developed by John Hastings, an editor at *Reader's Digest*, in collaboration with two registered dieticians and other weight-loss experts.

How does it work?
The key elements of the 12-week plan (which includes a "fast track" weight-loss option) are respecting portion sizes and eating healthily. The first four weeks focus on bringing about change in the dieter's life – one small step at a time. Week one focuses on improving breakfast, week two on improving lunch, week three on improving snacks and week four on improving dinner. The remaining eight weeks provide suggestions for dining at restaurants, during holidays, "fixing" the kitchen, self-assessment, managing stress, physical activity, relapse management and maintenance of the plan.

LONG-TERM PLAN

FLEXIBILITY

FAMILY FRIENDLY

COST

STRENGTH OF SCIENCE

sample menu
This plan focuses on making one beneficial

	saturday	sunday	monday	tuesday	
morning	100g low-fat cottage cheese, mini bagel, grapefruit sections	50g oat rings, 240ml 1% milk, raspberries	50g puffed wheat cereal, 240ml 1% milk, orange	mixed vegetable frittata, wholewheat toast, strawberries	
lunch	chef salad, 4 breadsticks, honeydew	ham sandwich, spinach-orange salad with apple and honey dressing, canteloupe	cheese sandwich, green salad with pecans, cider vinegar dressing, banana	plain burger, Caesar salad, watermelon	
supper	beef stroganoff, green beans, tomato slices in balsamic vinegar	grilled salmon, mesclun salad with palm hearts, grilled asparagus, dinner roll	scallops, angel hair pasta, cauliflower and broccoli, mixed greens	chicken breast, saffron rice, kidney beans, Brussels sprouts	
snack	ice fruit bar	jelly beans	nuts	microwave popcorn	

The book contains menus for a 1,300-calorie plan – a 300-calorie breakfast, 350-calorie lunch, 450-calorie dinner, and 200-calorie snacks – and information on modifying it to a 1,600-calorie plan.

Research supports the idea that a weight-loss plan focusing on a combination of portion control, eating management, and physical activity methods can be effective as a long-term weight-management strategy. The book and website (which provides an easy avenue for signing up to the programme and accessing its many services, such as recipes) are popular.

Pros and cons
The plan integrates change slowly, which may help the individual to learn and implement healthier behaviour patterns. The diet may result in a low calcium intake, so consultation with a qualified dietician may be required to plan a more adequate menu. Although the programme tries to avoid counting calories, it is in fact important to observe serving sizes to ensure an adherence to the given calorie limits.

Is it for you?
Not a "quick fix" to weight loss, this dieting model will appeal to those who want to shed the pounds by introducing changes slowly and managing not only what is eaten but also other factors which impact on eating behaviour. Although the plan has a calorie-balanced carbohydrate, protein and fat distribution that corresponds to the recommended amounts, everyone should consult a doctor before starting any diet programme. If you want to use the Change One principles but need a different calorie

healthy tips
- Suitable beverages include coffee or tea with a low-calorie creamer and artificial sweetener; lots of fluid – soda water, mineral water; diet colas; fruit juice (but fruit and water are better); one glass of wine or beer per day (about 100 calories).
- Nuts or seeds for a snack: 30 pistachios, a handful of pumpkin seeds, 10 peanuts, 16-20 almonds, 1 tablespoon of peanut butter.

intake from that used in the book, you may need to consult a dietician or nutritionist for guidance.

Availability
Most of the foods in the Change One Diet can be purchased from specialist food shops or supermarkets.

Lifestyle changes
The plan emphasizes the need for developing skills in order to manage certain eating situations such as snacking, eating out, creating a healthy "kitchen" environment, managing stress and relapse and incorporating physical activity.

change per week.

	wednesday	thursday	friday	**Resources**
	55g bulgar wheat cereal, 240ml 1% milk, apple	½ bagel, yogurt cheese*, yogurt with mango slices	80g wheat bran cereal, 240ml 1% milk, tangerine	www.changeone.com www.everydiet.org/change_one.htm **Hastings, J. *Change One* (2003, Reader's Digest)**
	vegetarian chili roll, spinach salad with low-fat dressing, blueberries	240ml beef barley soup, roll, turnip greens, orange	turkey sandwich, beetroot salad, sliced pineapple	
	grilled chicken, lettuce and tomato, wholewheat roll, coleslaw	kidney beans, rice, mixed baby greens, steamed carrots	grilled prawns, orzo pasta with peas and raisins, ratatouille	
	small soft pretzel	baked tortilla chips	low-fat brownie	

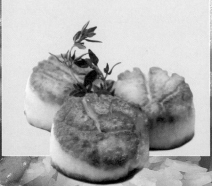

* **Recipe from Hastings, J. *Change One*.**

FRENCH WOMAN'S DIET

This non-diet focuses on a balanced relationship between eating and the pleasure derived from it, and advocates a lifelong strategy of quality over quantity, so you eat with your head, not your stomach.

LONG-TERM PLAN

FLEXIBILITY

FAMILY FRIENDLY

COST
●

STRENGTH OF SCIENCE

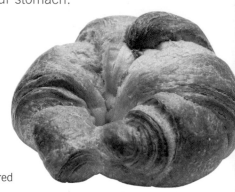

Diet history
This diet is based on the best-selling title *French Women Don't Get Fat: The Secret of Eating for Pleasure* (2005) by Mireille Guiliano.

How does it work?
Defined as a "comprehensive approach to living", the French Woman's Diet offers lifestyle strategies to women looking to lose up to 14kg (30lbs). The book is based on the experiences of the French-born-and-bred author now living in the United States.

Guiliano writes about the contrasting attitudes to food-related behaviour between French and American women from the angle of her own personal experience and observations. She proposes a four-phase plan to focus on "short-term recasting" (for about three months) as part of helping the dieter achieve a kind of mental French Zen.

Phase 1 is a three-week inventory of meals that acts as a wake-up call. It involves the individual evaluating his or her feeding habits to identify those foods that are being consumed excessively. This detailed assessment is conducted to identify specific situations which are provoking overeating in a person and to consider what types of food can be cut back or eliminated. The dieter is asked to reflect on the reasons he or she wants to lose weight and how current eating

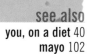

see also
you, on a diet 40
mayo 102

healthy tips
- Develop a personal culture of good habits. Eat three regular meals and go out for walks on a daily basis.
- Enjoy 100% natural bio-active yogurt. Buy or make your own – simply use fresh fruit or wheat germ as yummy toppings and drizzle on some honey.

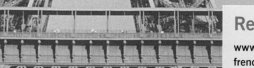

Resources

www.mireilleguiliano.com/frenchwomen.htm

diets.aol.com/a-z/french_women_diet_main

Guiliano, M. *French Women Don't Get Fat: The Secret of Eating for Pleasure* (2005, Random House)

patterns and food selections may be obstructing this goal.

Phase 2, part of the so-called process of recasting, can take from one to three months and involves a gradual dietary shift from quantity to quality. Individuals are advised not to rush this stage and indeed for some it may even take up to three months. During this time it is crucial to integrate a wide variety of foods into one's diet while cultivating attitudes and behaviour patterns that will enhance one's rate of success – for example, a positive approach to the rituals of grocery shopping and food preparation, a fondness for and regularity in drinking water, taking time to savour each meal, eating the appropriate portion sizes, refraining from stocking up on junk foods and coming up with suitable replacements to high-calorie foods.

Among the helpful suggestions on offer are ways of handling challenging situations, such as changing routes to avoid a particular trigger like a food shop. The plan advocates the avoidance of hunger through hunger management. This technique may include identifying small but satisfying snacks. Deprivation should not occur and occasionally planning to have favourite items, for example on the weekend, needs to be incorporated into the lifestyle plan.

When dining out, the focus should be on ordering small courses made with quality ingredients. The occasional glass of wine can be consumed as part of the meal.

Phase 3 involves stabilization but it is unclear just how separate it is from Phase 2. All types of food are re-introduced at this stage but in the appropriate amounts.

At Phase 4 the target weight has been achieved and the person's habits are now appropriate to their tastes and metabolic rate.

The plan makes the following basic recommendations:
1. Avoid the two extremes of either going hungry or feeling stuffed.
2. Avoid obsessing about eating and dieting.
3. Do not skip meals or deprive yourself of food.
4. Eat nuts as snacks or sprinkled over foods.
5. Eat real food in moderation instead of using substitutes.
6. Eat three daily meals that include carbohydrates, proteins and fats.
7. Do not replace regular meals with beverages such as shakes.
8. Eat yogurt with active cultures.
9. Eat without stuffing yourself or feeling guilty.
10. Enjoy high-quality bread and chocolate in moderate amounts.
11. Enjoy fresh foods and flavoursome fruits and vegetables in season.
12. Use either fresh or dried herbs and spices.
13. Focus on small portions of high-quality foods.
14. If you relapse, just get back on track.
15. Make physical activity an integral part of your day, starting with a "slow burn" approach in the form of dedicated daily walks and gradually building up to an increase in targeted movement (such as walking up a flight of stairs instead of using the lift). Use dumbbells to build up physical strength.
16. Plan what to eat in advance.
17. Savour meals, slow down, relax, and stop to eat – it is not part of multi-tasking.
18. Take pleasure in eating and focus on "good" not "bad" things to eat.

While not specific to this diet, the evidence indicates that behavioural approaches to weight loss which include portion control, regular physical activity, self-efficacy and self-regulation can be effective in long-term weight management.

Pros and cons

The French Woman's Diet focuses on developing an intelligent attitude to eating complemented by portion control for slow but permanent, long-term change. The downside is that the focus of this plan is on attitude and behavioural changes with no set structure, food prohibitions or structured meal patterns to follow.

Is it for you?

It is likely to appeal to those who do not like structured eating patterns and prefer a lifestyle-and-values approach. Anyone who needs guidance with what, when, where and how much to eat will find adhering to this plan challenging.

Availability

Nearly all the foods in this diet can be bought from any general food shop or supermarket.

Lifestyle changes

Although structured exercise is not strictly part of the plan, the person should partake in daily walking or other physical activities as part of a philosophy that is very much in the spirit of French living.

The diet advocates the "zip guide" as a self-regulating mechanism: rather than obsessing about weight, use the fit of your clothes as a guideline for changing your food habits or activity levels. Judge whether they fit comfortably, are a bit snug or very tight, and take action accordingly.

SCENTSATIONAL DIET

This unique "inhaler" plan promotes weight loss by using the smell of food to suppress appetite, increase satiety and control overeating impulses.

LONG-TERM PLAN

FLEXIBILITY

FAMILY FRIENDLY

COST

STRENGTH OF SCIENCE

Diet history

In 1996 Dr Alan R. Hirsh, a neurologist and psychiatrist from Cleveland Clinic Center in Ohio, observed that people with a temporary loss of smell (mostly due to medications) ate more and subsequently put on weight. When they recovered the use of their olfactory system, however, they resumed losing weight. This surprising discovery became the foundation of the unique Scentsational Diet.

How does it work?

The plan is based on the psychological-physiological dichotomy that "If I have smelled it, I have eaten it". As odour enters the nostrils during inhalation, the scent is intensified 1,000 times, causing the brain to send out the "stop eating" or satiety signal as a neurological message to the rest of the body triggering a sensation of fullness.

Apparently the more contact there is with a particular smell, the faster satiety levels are reached. The smell of hot food is released most efficiently of all to affect satisfaction levels quickly, but scientific

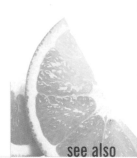

see also
nutrisystem 74

sample menu

Keep away from the buffet tables and salad

	saturday	sunday	monday	tuesday
morning	grapefruit, hummus with pitta bread, skimmed milk	hot green tea, bagel with flavoured cream cheese	hot chocolate, wheat flakes with skimmed milk, strawberries	orange juice, hot rice cereal, scrambled eggs
lunch	pepper steak with linguini, steamed marrow, apple slices	turkey sandwich with lettuce and tomato, green grapes, hot coffee	white rice with red beans, steamed green beans, orange juice	tuna salad wholemeal sandwich, steamed courgettes, cranberry juice
supper	baked potato with butter and minced meat, blueberry juice	broccoli cheese soup, breadcrumbs, mango slices	baked ham, mashed potatoes and carrot sticks, red grapes	meat burrito, green salad, skimmed milk
snack	kiwi fruit	peppermint ice cream	cranberry juice, peanut butter, Tuc biscuits	celery and carrot sticks

research indicating the part played by food odours in effective weight loss is still limited. A company called NutriSystem is now in the process of using this very principle to develop odour-infused, flavoured water that promotes weight loss.

Pros and cons

Easy to follow and involving pleasant smells, the Scentsational Diet also encourages the need for an exercise plan that will prompt faster weight loss. The downside is dieters' reliance on inhalers that emit the scents of certain types of foods – for example, sweet neutral scents such as green apples, bananas, and peppermint – to suppress appetite. Choosing different refills, however, may prevent monotony of smells.

The plan recommends avoiding buffet tables and salad bars because the variety of odours produced inhibits a person's ability to focus on one specific smell at a time to bring about a feeling of fullness or satiety. Most dairy products (including milk) should be reduced because the brain's satiety centre is not stimulated by their mild odor.

Is it for you?

Adults who need to lose only a small amount of weight (between 2kg and 7kg (5–15lb) may not find the Scentsational Diet especially helpful but the plan is definitely not suited to people with allergies, sinus problems, asthma or recurrent nasal congestion.

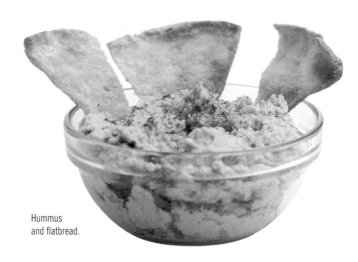

Hummus and flatbread.

Availability

All foods in this diet are widely available but those with naturally sweet aromas are favoured. Choose hot, aromatic foods (soups, coffee, chocolate and teas) and spicy dishes for curbing hunger pangs.

Lifestyle changes

Get used to sniffing sweet neutral scents (such as green apples, bananas and peppermint) before eating, chew well, eat slowly and opt for hot, spicy foods. Keep away from salad bars and dairy foods.

bars and limit dairy foods.

wednesday	thursday	friday	Resources
hot apple cider, chocolate puffed cereal, tangerine	banana, porridge with skimmed milk, boiled egg	green apple muffin with cinnamon, coffee with cream substitute and sweetener	www.scentsationalhealth.com www.ScentSationalTechnologies.com
chili with cream crackers, celery sticks, fresh fruit salad with cream cheese	Southwestern chicken salad, pomegranate juice	minestrone soup, baked salmon and boiled potatoes, honeydew slices	Hirsch, A. R. *Scentsational Weight Loss: At Last a New Easy Natural Way To Control Your Appetite* (1997, Element Books)
roasted chicken breast, wild rice and beans, fresh spinach, orange juice	cabbage soup, sirloin steak with mushroom sauce, tomato juice	wholewheat spaghetti with meatballs, steamed vegetables, skimmed milk	
Digestive biscuits, grape juice	dark chocolate chip cookies, green apple juice	orange sections	

Note: This diet does not provide a specific menu.

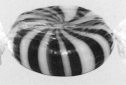

Treat yourself to peppermint candy in small amounts.

LONG-TERM PLAN

●●●

FLEXIBILITY

●●

FAMILY FRIENDLY

●●●

COST

●

STRENGTH OF SCIENCE

●●●

SUPERMARKET DIET

This balanced guide to eating focuses on nutritious supermarket foods and includes three menu categories: 1,200 calories (Boot Camp), 1,500 calories (Keep on Losing) and 1,800 calories (Stay Slim Maintenance).

Diet history

Endorsed by the popular monthly US women's magazine, *Good Housekeeping*'s Supermarket Diet also recently appeared in a book by a registered dietician. Based on the scientific evidence related to nutrition and the selection of foods, it is relatively new and not yet well known so is likely to grow in popularity.

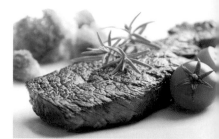

How does it work?

The rationale behind the plan combines a low-calorie intake through controlled dieting along with an increased expenditure of energy from regular exercise. The book provides a body of detailed information for following this diet carefully, including tips on how to shop, read labels and select ingredients. Forbidden foods are high in fat or sugar, "empty" calories, and highly sweetened beverages while high-fibre, low-calorie vegetables and fruits are encouraged as "treats".

The gradual step-by-step guide is designed to convert the dieter to a new eating programme and encourages a lifestyle plan to bring on

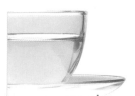

see also
mediterranean 160
mypyramid 162

sample menu

This diet is designed to convert the dieter to a

	saturday	sunday	monday	tuesday
morning	hot cereal, milk, fruit, nuts, coffee or tea	fruit-topped waffles, milk, drink	strawberry smoothie, toast, coffee	bran muffin, fruit, milk, coffee or tea
lunch	tomato soup, tuna and cannellini bean salad, drink	mushroom soup, Waldorf salad with turkey, drink	baked potato and chilli, salad, fruit, tea	cafeteria meal, salad bar, fruit, drink
supper	grilled halibut, baked potato, vegetables, tossed salad, yogurt, drink	filet mignon, grilled tomatoes, mashed potatoes, sugar-snap peas, spinach salad	burger in a bun, boiled potatoes, carrots, green beans, green salad, drink	roast chicken, brown rice, stir-fried cougette, onion and mushrooms, spinach salad with nuts or fruit
snack 1	low-fat chocolate milk, biscuit	wholewheat crackers with smoked salmon	plain yogurt, apple	low-fat frozen yogurt
snack 2	salted mixed nuts	fat-free popcorn, yogurt	mixed nuts	fruit and nuts

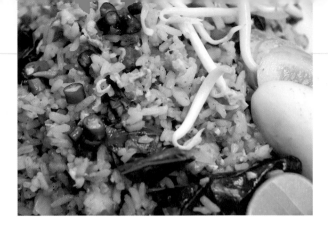

Stir-fried vegetables with brown rice and small amounts of a monounsaturated oil like peanut oil.

weight loss and instil healthy eating habits. The Supermarket Diet involves staying away from food and lifestyle choices that may cause weight gain.

The first two weeks of the 1,200-calorie Boot Camp menu offer a sensible kick-start to weight loss. The second and third stages of this low-calorie, high-fibre, low-fat and low-sugar plan ease the individual into responsible eating habits and physical activities based on gender and weight in order to reach the desired goal while keeping hunger at bay. There are various easy-to-prepare menus, family meal suggestions and handy grocery shopping tips.

Pros and cons
A practical, science-based and straightforward approach to weight loss, the Supermarket Diet provides common-sense guidelines for following a healthy lifestyle and not just a temporary fad. The exchange lists introduced to regulate both portion size and the number of calories include meals that do not require lengthy preparation

(5–20 minutes) yet still offer variety and a balance of nutrients. The programme is proof that you can stock the larder with nutritious foods and cook a meal the whole family will enjoy. As a minus, however, patience and perseverance are necessary as results are not immediate.

Is it for you?
The Supermarket Diet will appeal to individuals wanting a balanced approach to maintaining a healthy weight. Children can follow this regime if the meals and portions are suitable for their age.

Availability
All foods in this diet are available from any general food shop or supermarket. The meal suggestions are inexpensive choices and mostly homecooked.

Lifestyle changes
This plan emphasizes the need for regular exercise and the adoption of healthy behavioural changes.

forbidden foods
- chips and fried snacks
- fatty dips
- doughnuts
- biscuits and crackers
- sugary drinks
- honey, jams and jellies
- cream or butter-iced cakes
- ice cream
- all kinds of sweets

free foods
- very low-calorie or calorie-free foods and beverages

new eating plan with a lifestyle change.

wednesday	thursday	friday
peach smoothie, toast, coffee or tea	cold cereal, milk, fruit, coffee or tea	eggs, toast, milk, fruit, coffee or tea
lentil soup, spinach salad with fruit, toast, coffee	toasted cheese sandwich, chicken salad, drink	vegetable soup, chickpea salad, toast, drink
grilled steak (orange-glazed steak), sweet potato, asparagus, cauliflower, Caesar salad, drink	grilled salmon (with honey-lime glaze), garlic bread, broccoli, green beans, spring mix salad with nuts	chicken with couscous and spinach, tabbouleh salad, hummus and pitta toasts, drink
fruit yogurt, biscuit	wholewheat crackers, cream cheese	apple, cheddar cheese
pretzels, milk	low-fat flavoured yogurt	frozen yogurt, crackers

Resources
www.msnbc.msn.com/id/16694314

Jibrin, J. *Good Housekeeping Book, The Supermarket Diet* (2007, Hearst/ Sterling Publishing)

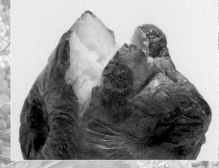

Note: The number of calories vary according to each stage. Plans for the diet's three stages are given as examples. *Jibrin, J. *The Supermarket Diet*.

LONG-TERM PLAN

FLEXIBILITY

FAMILY FRIENDLY

COST

STRENGTH OF SCIENCE

THE ULTIMATE NEW YORK DIET

A three-phase eight-week "eating, exercising and thinking plan" for shedding pounds that focuses on teaching results that can be maintained for a lifetime.

Diet history

The plan was developed by David Kirsch, author of *The Ultimate New York Body Plan* (2004) and founder and owner of Madison Square Club, a fitness training club in New York City specializing in customized fitness training.

How does it work?

Nutritionally this three-phase plan takes a low-carb, high-protein approach. Phase One is the strictest and forbids foods from six lists called A, B, C, D, E and F, but includes some protein shakes. It eliminates breads or other starches, dairy, sweet foods, fruits, most fats and alcohol. Recommended as a two-week phase (or longer) in order to achieve the weight-loss goal, the Phase One plan is a combination of strict dieting and 45 to 90 minutes of daily exercise, some of which requires a medicine ball or dumbbells and can be done either in one go or separately in

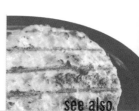

see also
you, on a diet 40
south beach 64

sample menu

This is a sample Phase One menu plan, which

	saturday	sunday	monday	tuesday
morning	David's Protein Meal-Replacement Shake*	David's Protein Meal-Replacement Shake*	David's Protein Meal-Replacement Shake*	David's Protein Meal-Replacement Shake*
lunch	roast turkey, Brussels sprouts, mixed greens	chicken breast with Mexican salsa, steamed spinach, mixed greens	chicken breast, steamed spinach, mixed greens	turkey meatloaf, steamed broccoli, mixed greens
supper	David's Protein Meal-Replacement Shake*	grilled halibut, steamed spinach, green salad	turkey chilli, cauliflower mash, green salad	David's Protein Meal-Replacement Shake*
snack 1	salmon burger	egg white and turkey scramble	10 raw almonds	hard-boiled egg whites
snack 2	turkey burger	10 raw almonds	chunky light tuna	10 raw almonds

ten-minute mini sessions. Phase Two adds back one carbohydrate serving per day as part of the mid-morning snack or lunch. The book provides four weeks' worth of menus for Phase Three but it is intended to be a lifelong plan. Phase One and Phase Two are basically low-calorie, low-carbohydrate programmes. Phase Three includes menus but has some meals known as "cheat meals" that allow a glass of wine. Without these kinds of meals, Phase Three plans too are low in calories but the total intake will vary depending on the calories of the "cheat meal".

Pros and cons

The plan provides a highly structured approach to diet, weight loss and exercise. It includes the weight reduction and weight stabilization components that many other quick-fix plans lack. This strict low-carbohydrate, low-calorie plan, however, may be challenging for some dieters and the exercise regimen demanding for individuals without the adequate initial level of physical fitness. Overextending Phase One could eventually result in inadequate calcium, vitamin A and vitamin C levels

weigh this up...

Phase One prohibited foods:
A = alcohol
B = bread
C = starchy carbohydrates and coffee
D = dairy
E = extra sweets
F = fruits and most fats

Phase One approved snacks:
tuna in spring water
tinned wild salmon
hard-boiled egg whites
scrambled egg whites
raw almonds

plus a low intake of other vitamins and minerals.

Is it for you?

This plan will appeal to persons who like low-carbohydrate meals and a structured diet and exercise phased approach to pound shedding and weight management. Persons who need to restrict their physical activity for medical reasons or who have special conditions need to consult a doctor beforehand.

Availability

Many of the foods in this diet can be purchased in a general food shop or supermarket but some of the turkey-based products will require some searching. The whey protein powder needed for the protein shakes may require shopping at a specialist food shop.

Lifestyle changes

The plan includes physical activity as part of its weight-loss strategy.

Asian pepper chicken.

includes meal-replacement shakes.

wednesday	thursday	friday
egg whites with shiitake mushrooms	David's Protein Meal-Replacement Shake*	egg whites with minced turkey and tomatoes
grilled salmon, steamed asparagus, mixed greens	David's Protein Meal-Replacement Shake*	turkey meatloaf, vegetable caponata, mixed greens
turkey salad, steamed cauliflower, mixed greens, tomatoes	David's Protein Meal-Replacement Shake*	Asian pepper chicken*, bok choy, green salad
grilled salmon	turkey burger	10 raw almonds
scrambled egg whites	10 raw almonds	scrambled egg whites

Resources

http://davidkirsch.co.uk

www.weightlossresources.co.uk/diet/reviews/new_york_body_plan.htm

Kirsch, D. *The Ultimate New York Diet* (2006, McGraw Hill)

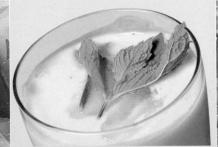

* The recipe for David's Protein Meal-Replacement Shake and recipes for dishes similar to those in this plan are available in the book, *The Ultimate New York Diet*.

LONG-TERM PLAN

FLEXIBILITY

FAMILY FRIENDLY
●●

COST
●

STRENGTH OF SCIENCE

YOU, ON A DIET

A lifestyle dietary plan that emphasizes "waist-not-weight" changes.

Diet history

The plan was developed by Dr Roizen and Dr Oz, authors of *You, The Owner's Manual* (2005), *You, On a Diet* (2006) and *You, The Smart Patient* (2006). The focus of *You, On a Diet* and *You, The Owner's Manual* are on helping the reader understand the human body.

How does it work?

The plan includes three main meals and foods rich in fibre to help stop cravings. The one-week "rebooting" or start-up plan lasts two weeks and focuses on eating the same or similar kinds of food (for example, dry wholegrain cereal for breakfast on most days). Among the usual foods prescribed are whole grains, nuts, fruits, vegetables, lean meats (if preferred, it is possible to opt for poultry over beef) and fish. The diet recommends 10 tablespoons of cooked tomato sauce a week as well as a daily multivitamin supplement.

The book discusses how the body stores and burns fat, why waist size is more indicative of general health than overall weight and how to develop a regular physical activity programme to suit you. Emphasis is placed on the importance of daily exercise, including walking, stretching and muscle-strengthening workouts three times a week.

The diet emphasizes regular calorie-controlled eating using foods that are healthy, recommends daily physical activity, and suggests behavioural strategies for addressing hunger, relapse, dining out and other dieting pitfalls. The book includes a one-week menu and a shopping list for staples.

see also
good-carb low-carb 62
sonoma 104

sample menu

Repetition in weeks

	saturday	sunday	monday	tuesday
morning	high-fibre wholegrain cereal, 120ml calcium-fortified soya milk, fruit	pineapple-banana smoothie with soya powder	porridge, 120ml skimmed milk, fruit	omelette with 3 egg whites, mixed vegetables
lunch	Caesar salad, grilled chicken, low-calorie dressing	tomato lentil soup, carrot and celery sticks	meal-sized green salad, 110g fish	mixed vegetable soup, cos lettuce and tomato salad
supper	grilled fish, steamed mixed vegetables, tomato juice	cos lettuce salad, grilled chicken strips	tofu and bean chilli in tomato sauce, brown rice, orange juice* spritzer	wholewheat pizza with veggie topping, grapefruit juice*
snack 1	2 kiwi fruit	orange	low-fat yogurt with fresh berries	baked cinnamon apple
snack 2	pear, low-fat yogurt	plain popcorn, sparkling water	plain popcorn, sparkling water	30g raw almonds

Baked cinnamon apple is an easy-to-make dessert.

treats
PICK FROM:
- You Soup (from the book)
- vegetables
- edamame (fresh soya beans)
- wholewheat

- pitta toast
- baked apples
- low-fat yogurt
- sugar-free gum
- almonds

Pros and cons
This short-term diet incorporates a one-week plan that the dieter puts together from the variety of options provided and then repeats for a second week. Although the duration is short, the plan must be carried out twice.

Is it for you?
This eating programme will appeal to people who are interested in knowing how their body functions, how waist size relates to weight management and those searching for a lifestyle approach to weight loss. Individuals with limitations as regards any form of physical exercise must consult a doctor before beginning any of the activities in the plan.

Availability
All the foods in this diet can be readily purchased from any general food shop or supermarket.

Lifestyle changes
Daily physical activity is an integral part of the plan and several behaviour management techniques are also used.

weigh this up...
- If you relapse, do not give up. Simply re-focus on your goals to get you back on track.

one and two helps with planning.

wednesday	thursday	friday
high-fibre wholegrain cereal, 120ml skimmed milk or fortified soya milk, fruit	porridge, 120ml skimmed milk, fruit	2 scrambled eggs, turkey sausage
meal-sized green salad, 110g grilled chicken	veggie burger on wholewheat bread, spinach salad	meal-sized green salad, 110g grilled turkey
roasted chicken, stewed tomatoes, sparkling water	grilled ginger salmon, brown rice, sparkling water	pasta primavera, grape juice spritzer
plum	plain popcorn, sparkling water	low-fat yogurt smoothie with strawberries
low-fat yogurt with fresh berries	baked apple	55g wholegrain cereal and raisins

* Use calcium-fortified juices.

Resources
www.realage.com/doctorCenter/YouOnADiet

Roizen, M.F., Oz, M.C. *You, On a Diet* (2005, Simon & Schuster)

ATKINS DIET

Although this low-carbohydrate, high-fat, high-protein classic eating plan has fluctuated in popularity over the years, it continues to influence a range of similar diets.

Diet history

Using low- or non-carbohydrate diets for rapid weight loss can be traced back to the 1800s but the origins of this practice probably date back to an even earlier time.

The Atkins Diet first became popular during the 1960s when clinically obese individuals were admitted to a hospital for medical treatment. Physicians tried reducing patients' weight by temporarily omitting carbohydrates from their diet to treat related diseases.

Published in the early 1990s, *Dr Atkins' New Diet Revolution* became a bestseller overnight and numerous media stories – some favourable, some not – started to circulate. The most recent Atkins plan promotes five different nutritional "rules": a high consumption of protein, fibre, substantial vitamin and mineral intake, the elimination of trans fats and low amounts of sugar. Although physical activity is encouraged alongside the diet plan, the main focus is on the high-protein, low-carbohydrate regime.

Before scientific data existed, a combination of consumer interest, well-timed marketing strategies and shrewd media coverage

LONG-TERM PLAN

FLEXIBILITY

FAMILY FRIENDLY

COST

STRENGTH OF SCIENCE

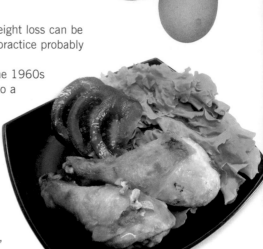

see also
south beach 64

sample menu
Menus consist of a variety of meats or fish with

	saturday	sunday	monday	tuesday
morning	courgette, red peppers, and apricot juice, baked eggs and pancetta, coffee or tea	cherry and apple juice, bacon and asparagus frittata, tea or coffee	mixed vegetable juice, egg or bacon, cheese, coffee or tea	tomato, carrot and red pepper juice, ham, tomato, sautéed mushrooms, tea/coffee
snack	Turkish spinach dip with vegetables	Peking duck wraps	broccoli and cauliflower with cream cheese	celery, peanut butter
lunch	fish cakes with herbs, roasted Mediterranean vegetables	pork and peach salad, stir-fried aubergine, tofu	roast beef, green beans, carrots, green salad	veal cutlet, Greek salad, grilled butternut squash, green beans
snack	smoked salmon cones	Denver omelette	cheese snack	cottage cheese, peaches
dinner	grilled pork chops, baby beetroot salad, lettuce wedges	grilled turkey kebabs, chicory and grapefruit salad	fried fish, marrow, courgette and red pepper frittata, Caesar salad	grilled white fish, bacon and asparagus frittata, green salad

catapulted this diet into the limelight and sealed its popularity. The Atkins Corporation today promotes not only the Atkins Diet but also a wide range of branded products including foods and supplements designed to be consumed as part of the plan. Consumers can subscribe to websites and clubs, receive newsletters, download recipes, participate in discussion groups and even take courses on the subject.

Low-carbohydrate diet plans have turned up under many different names and been marketed by different promoters over the years. Dr Robert C. Atkins, the most famous of its advocates, published *The Atkins No Carbohydrate Diet* in 1972. The original diet was extremely limited in terms of food choice and was later modified to include fruits and vegetables. Following a dip in popularity and a few more modifications, consumer interest was renewed but the Atkins Diet remains controversial to this day.

Another variation of the low-carb plan is the South Beach Diet which has gained recent popularity and includes fruit, vegetables, limited grains and transitional phases. Many overweight and obese individuals use low-carb diets to shed unwanted weight fast. Although initially this is water weight, it may provide motivation to continue.

These days "Atkins" and "low carbohydrate" are terms synonymous with carbohydrate limitation and a high protein intake (usually accompanied by high fat) from meat, fish and other sources. Due in large part to the protein and fat, this diet has found favour with the general public because individuals feel satisfied or full for longer than on other diets.

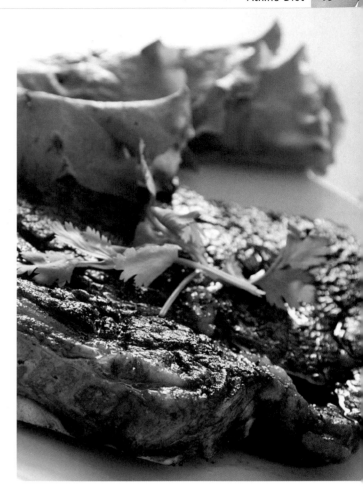

vegetables to control carbohydrate intake.

wednesday	thursday	friday
tomato and spinach juice, smoked salmon omelette, coffee or tea	cucumber, celery and apple juice, tomato and eggs on corn tortilla, coffee or tea	carrot juice, scrambled eggs with dill and smoked salmon, tea or coffee
mozzarella, tomatoes	celery and tomato salsa, cheese sticks	carrot broccoli and cauliflower, cheese dip
grilled vegetables and ricotta steak, lettuce wedges	mixed vegetable pesto, tuna Caesar salad with nuts	beef and sweetcorn soup, Reuben salad, mixed nuts
corn tortilla, cheese	herbed olive, white beans and anchovy dip	Japanese chicken skewers
sweet and sour grilled chicken, mixed vegetables, salad	rosemary lamb roast, roasted butternut squash, bacon and feta frittata	braised cornish hens, Brussels sprouts, creamed spinach

Resources

www.atkins.com

www.atkinsexposed.org/atkins

Atkins. R. *Dr. Atkins' New Diet Revolution* (2002, HarperCollins)

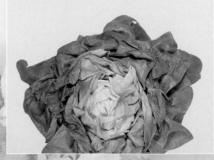

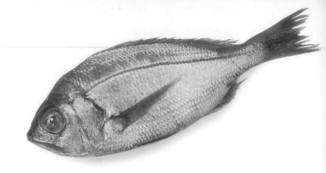

How does it work?

The Atkins Diet recommends a restricted amount of carbohydrate intake for the first couple of weeks during the Induction Phase, then gradually introduces an increased amount of carbohydrates. During the Maintenance Phase, carbohydrates are allowed to be eaten in small amounts to control the release of insulin.

A limited carbohydrate intake will trigger a state of starvation in the body because the brain, nervous system and blood depend on the glucose obtained from carbohydrates for optimal functioning.

When food intake fails to provide the minimum amount of carbohydrate required, the body resorts to breaking down proteins from muscle and body fat reserves to obtain glucose for energy. Any proteins or fats left over are broken down into ketones – substances which must be purged by the kidneys.

Dehydration may occur because these substances are eliminated or washed out using water from the body's tissues.

The Atkins Diet causes the rapid shedding of pounds largely from water lost by the kidneys, with some burning of fat. To minimize loss of body water and to help flush out ketones, a high consumption of water is strongly recommended.

A long-term study on Atkins reported the greatest loss early on, with no significant results by those on a low-carbohydrate versus a low-fat diet at the end of one year.

Whether following Atkins or a similar plan, remember that low-carbohydrate diets generally last for a short period of time. When used for extreme obesity, they should be monitored by a doctor or registered dietician. Medical supervision is key so dehydration levels and excess ketones can be kept under control.

Low-carbohydrate diets are usually recommended for up to three or four weeks because longer durations may cause serious side effects.

Pros and cons

The Atkins Corporation promotes a whole range of products that are complementary to the plan but in no way integral to following the diet successfully. The Atkins Diet causes rapid initial weight loss and may be effective for kick-starting any weight-loss regime.

Short-term research studies tracking the progress of individuals on the diet have reported high levels of satiety, a temporary improvement in lipid levels or glucose stability in the

weigh this up...
• Without any carbohydrates in your diet, your body will break down proteins and fats for energy to produce acidic substances called ketones.

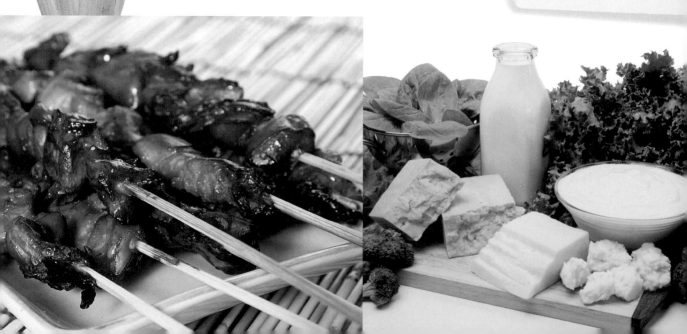

bloodstream, some loss of body fat, and the sparing of body protein.

There are as yet no findings available beyond one year. Long-term data is difficult to obtain, and information on the extended consequences of the diet is not known because subjects find it challenging to remain on this type of diet for extended lengths of time.

Before beginning the Atkins Plan, it is important to consider the following possible consequences:

- Dehydration: if prolonged, a considerable loss of water is not beneficial to the body.
- Loss of calcium: if prolonged, bones become brittle which could help accelerate osteoporosis.
- Kidney problems: these organs may become stressed in trying to eliminate ketones from the body's system.
- Blood ketone levels: in excess, their presence results in the overproduction of uric acid, a risk factor in gout (painful swelling of the joints) and kidney stones.
- Digestive problems: a dietary lack of fibre obtained from foods such as whole grains, vegetables and fruit may disrupt regulation of the digestive system and indirectly cause constipation, diverticulosis and other intestinal problems.
- Changes in blood lipids: the data indicate short-term improvement in low density lipoproteins (LDL), cholesterol and triglycerides but nothing is known about the long-term effects.
- Limited food choice: dietary boredom could cause the weight lost to pile back on once the diet is stopped.
- Feelings of deprivation: many people find it almost impossible to reduce let alone give up rice, bread, cereals, pasta, fruits and sweets.

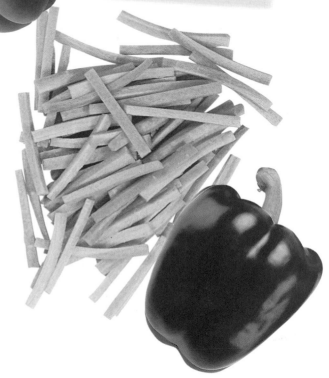

healthy tips
During the plan:
- Drink plenty of water
- Select lean meat and fish
- Eat lots of vegetables
- Have regular medical checkups.

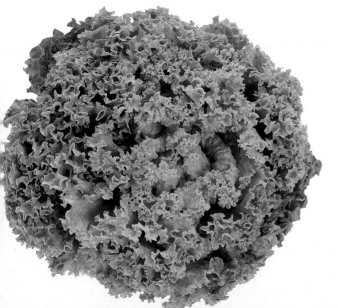

Is it for you?
Teenagers, anyone with kidney, heart or circulation problems, or special medical conditions should consult a doctor.

Availability
Atkins products range from breakfast bars, shakes, supplements and sweets to software and books. They are readily available from many general food shops or supermarkets.

Lifestyle changes
The newer version of the diet recommends about 30 minutes of daily exercise (such as aerobics and weightlifting), especially when experiencing a weight-loss plateau where stabilization has occurred.

LONG-TERM PLAN

●●●

FLEXIBILITY

●●

FAMILY FRIENDLY

●●●

COST

●

STRENGTH OF SCIENCE

●●

COMPLETE HIP AND THIGH DIET

This low-fat diet is moderately high in carbohydrates and proteins and specifically targets weight reduction from the hip and thigh area.

Diet history
Rosemary Conley wrote *The Hip and Thigh Diet* (1988) followed by *The Complete Hip and Thigh Diet* (1989).

How does it work?
The Complete Hip and Thigh Diet is based on the rationale that a regulated eating programme works because it prevents the kind of impulsive bingeing which results from overly restricted diets and severe calorie counting.

Breakfast consists of cereal, fruit, lean meat, fish or poultry accompanied by vegetables. Lunchtime meals include fruit, sandwiches, meat or seafood salads, soup or vegetables (including potatoes if desired). Dinner allows fruit, vegetables, soup, lean meat, fish or poultry, pasta, and you can have sorbet or yogurt for dessert.

The recommended daily requirements are 240–360ml of skimmed or low-fat milk, a minimum of 350g of fruit, 170g of protein, 350g of vegetables, 170g of grains, 140g of low-fat yogurt and fruit juice in moderation. Red meat is limited to two helpings a week. A typical meal includes lean meat, poultry, legumes, moderate amounts of

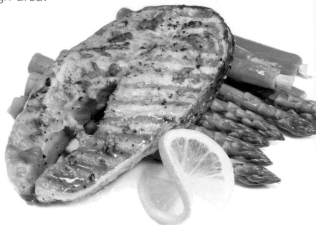

Baked or grilled fish and vegetables make a good midday meal.

see also
ultimate new york 38
you, on a diet 40

sample menu
This diet offers selections from a wide variety of

	saturday	sunday	monday	tuesday
morning	1 whole (170g) grapefruit, 140g yogurt	30g very lean bacon, 110g mushrooms, 140g yogurt, 120ml peach nectar	4 wholewheat crackers, 120ml skimmed milk	110g peaches canned in fruit juice, 140g yogurt
lunch	120ml skimmed milk, 360ml vegetable soup, 6 wholegrain crackers	170g baked chicken breast, 170g grapes, 120ml skimmed milk	120ml skimmed milk, fruit salad, 350g lettuce with kidney beans and sweetcorn	120ml skimmed milk, 110g plums, 120g tuna salad, 4 rye crackers
supper	120ml skimmed milk, 170g haddock poached in white wine, 170g plums	170g cooked pasta, 230g tinned tomatoes, 2 apples, 120ml skimmed milk	140g yogurt, 110g citrus fruit cup, 2 slices wholegrain bread	lettuce salad with tomatoes, onions, celery, cucumber and dressing, 1 apple, 120ml skimmed milk

starchy carbohydrate and an unrestricted intake of vegetables. Testimonials are used to support the claim that the weight loss is targeted and designed to come off mostly from the thighs and hips. Although the scientific evidence does support the usefulness of a moderate- to high-carbohydrate, moderate-protein, and low-fat diet for long-term weight loss, there is a lack of data to uphold the idea that a low-fat diet can specifically target weight loss around the hips and thighs.

Pros and cons
With careful planning and monitoring, this kind of eating regime can turn out to be nutritionally balanced in spite of its restriction on nuts, seeds and some dairy products. The diet, however, may be low in healthy fats.

An overabundance of testimonials would seem to support the diet's claims but there is an absence of scientific findings to give credence to the assertion that by following this specific diet the weight comes off the hips and thighs specifically.

Is it for you?
This diet is likely to appeal to people who are tired of calorie counting and fed up with eating programmes that advise a very restricted food intake.

It has been suggested that the Complete Hip and Thigh Diet would be helpful for binge sufferers. Anyone with an eating disorder, including binge eating, however, should seek professional advice from a qualified nutrition professional (such as a registered dietician) and a doctor rather than rely on testimonials alone.

Availability
All foods in this diet are widely available from any grocery shop or general supermarket

Lifestyle changes
Regular exercise is recommended as part of the plan.

forbidden foods
- margarine
- cream
- oil and fried foods
- fatty fish and meat
- poultry skin
- cheese and egg products
- egg yolk
- nuts
- sunflower seeds
- avocados
- ice cream and puddings
- chocolate

free foods
- cucumber
- celery
- carrots
- tomatoes
- peppers
- potatoes without any added fat
- unsweetened tea or black coffee (or with some skimmed milk allowance)

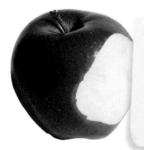

healthy tips
- Select low-fat yogurts and add fruit. This is often fewer calories than a commercial yogurt.

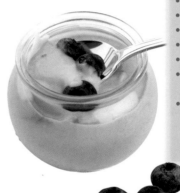

foods but limits red meat.

wednesday	thursday	friday
55g lean ham, 2 tomatoes, 1 wholewheat roll, 120ml skimmed milk	55g wholewheat cereal, 120ml skimmed milk, 120ml orange juice	5 stewed prunes, 2 slices wholegrain toast, 1 teaspoon orange marmalade, 120ml skimmed milk
2 boiled potatoes, 140g yogurt, 2 oranges, sliced	170g baked beans, 120ml skimmed milk, 350g pineapple	230g fresh fruit salad, 140g yogurt
baked cod with 110g brown rice, pears stuffed with cottage cheese, 120ml skimmed milk	1 baked potato, 170g sliced skinless turkey served with cranberries, 140g yogurt	170g beef strips, stir-fry vegetables, couscous, 120ml skimmed milk, orange

Resources
www.annecollins.com

www.skinnyondiets.com

Conley, R. *The Complete Hip and Thigh Diet* (1989, Warner Books)

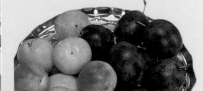

Note: All yogurt is low fat/low calorie. All salad dressings are reduced oil.

LONG-TERM PLAN

FLEXIBILITY

FAMILY FRIENDLY

COST

STRENGTH OF SCIENCE

DEAN ORNISH DIET

This low-fat vegetarian plan includes complex carbohydrates such as grains, fruit and vegetables. As well as promoting weight loss, it may also help to counteract the risk of cardiovascular disease.

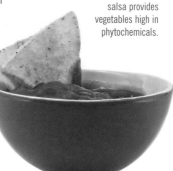

Baked tortilla chips are low in fat, and salsa provides vegetables high in phytochemicals.

Diet history
Dean Ornish is a cardiologist and Clinical Professor of Medicine at San Francisco's University of California. Since the 1990s, his numerous studies and scientific publications have shown that cardiovascular disease can be reversed, health improved and the body's excess fat stores reduced by a change of lifestyle and diet. His book *Eat More, Weigh Less* was featured on the *New York Times* bestseller list in 2002.

How does it work?
Based on vegetarian principles, this cardiovascular-reversible weight-loss programme advocates the consumption of whole foods, complex carbohydrates and a variety of fruit and vegetables for the recommended amount of carbohydrates and proteins. The foods in the plan provide adequate energy and the required bulk so the rate of metabolism does not slow down and hunger pangs are not felt.

Only 10 per cent of the total number of calories (energy) are from fats, which makes the diet very restrictive. It also limits simple forms

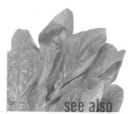

see also
pritikin 58

sample menu
This plan offers heart disease protection but

	saturday	sunday	monday	tuesday	
morning	apple, walnut and cinnamon muffins, fruit yogurt, tofu, jam, peaches, warm beverage	egg-white vegetable omelette, soya milk, fresh fruit salad, toast, warm beverage	cereal, yogurt, toast, berries, orange juice, warm beverage	cinnamon-raisin porridge, milk, toast, jam, warm beverage	
lunch	couscous salad, roasted aubergine, cucumber, onion, tomato and herb salad, fresh fruit, hot tea	pasta, mixed vegetable salad with ginger dressing, onion soup with tofu, bread, fruit, tea	baked potato, broccoli, olive and chickpea salad, lemon tarragon dressing, tossed green salad, fresh fruit, iced tea	mixed green salad, hummus, tabbouleh, bread, baked butternut squash, fresh fruit salad, water	
supper	basmati rice, grilled tofu, mixed green salad, creamed carrot, peas, cauliflower, dried fruit	vegetables: potato, aubergine, green beans, peas, courgettes and tomato sauce, cabbage and broccoli or cauliflower nut salad, bread	sun-dried tomato bruschetta, pasta with red peppers, greens and haricot beans, grilled asparagus with red peppers, fruit with nuts	rice with okra and tomatoes, steamed green pepper with onion, beetroot and broccoli, greens, baked pears with raisins, fruit salad	
snack 1	melon balls	dried fruit mix	baby carrots	baked crisps, salsa	
snack 2	yogurt	peaches	apple	banana nut bread	

of carbohydrates such as sugar and honey. The restriction on fats and simple sugars prevents individuals consuming excess calories, and the high fibre content helps satiety.

There is strong scientific evidence to support the plan's claim of reversing the risk of coronary artery disease. The resulting weight loss is due to the low caloric intake.

Pros and cons

In addition to weight loss, the Dean Ornish Diet promotes a healthy heart plus high intake of phytochemicals from vegetarian-based foods. However, it is more restrictive than a standard vegetarian diet. Meat-eaters accustomed to a typical Western diet might not adapt easily.

Is it for you?

Vegetarians, semi-vegetarians and anyone who likes a wide variety of foods and preparations will enjoy this diet. The programme is easy to follow for those who can go without meat and fried foods, including vegetarians, health-conscious individuals and lovers of whole foods. If planned carefully, a vegetarian-style plan will be less expensive than a regular diet because good-quality meat is often one of the most expensive ingredients to buy.

Growing children, especially young girls, should avoid this diet. Women planning to become or who are pregnant, adults with some types of anaemia or osteoporosis, and people who require a low potassium intake should consult their doctor beforehand. When on the diet, be sure to take enough iron, calcium, zinc and vitamin B12 supplements.

weigh this up...
- The restriction on fats from nuts and fish might work well for the reversal of coronary artery disease but these sources are essential for good health as they contain essential Omega-3 fatty acids.

Availability

All the foods in this diet are available from regular food shops and no special or exotic foods are recommended.

Lifestyle changes

This weight-loss plan advocates a comprehensive lifestyle change, including stress management training, stopping smoking, meditation and moderate exercise.

free foods
- cucumbers
- celery
- spinach
- greens
- some salad vegetables

forbidden foods
- fats and oils
- nuts
- seeds
- avocados
- white flour
- white rice

requires significant lifestyle changes.

wednesday	thursday	friday
fruit pancake, fresh berries, plain yogurt, toast, jam, warm beverage	apple and cranberry muffins, soya milk, fresh fruit compote, warm beverage	scrambled tofu, toast, jam, yogurt, fresh melon and berries, warm beverage
grilled vegetable wraps, thin bread, mixed bean soup, cantaloupe, orange, herb tea	haricot beans, greens and sun-dried tomatoes,crostini, black bean soup, tossed green salad, banana, hot tea	Italian bean salad, black pepper polenta, red pepper sauce, shiitake mushrooms, green salad, fruit gelatine
Spanish rice, strawberry, walnut and spinach salad, snap beans, peas, cauliflower and onion, grilled pineapple	spinach ravioli, tomato sauce, split pea and lentil soup, green salad with ginger dressing, baked apples with raisins	vegetable lasagne, grilled aubergine, courgettes, onion and green peppers, Caesar salad with vinegar dressing, croutons, fruit compote
peaches and berries	celery and creamed tofu	grapes and nuts
yogurt, carrots	oranges	banana

Resources

www.ornish.com

Ornish, D. *Eat More, Weigh Less* (2002, Quill, HarperCollins)

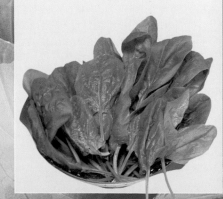

**Note: The sample menu is a vegetarian adaptation of the plan in *Eat More, Weigh Less*. All yogurt is fat free.
All breads are wholewheat and all grains are whole grain, including brown rice and wholewheat pasta.**

LONG-TERM PLAN

FLEXIBILITY

FAMILY FRIENDLY

COST

STRENGTH OF SCIENCE

GLYCAEMIC INDEX (GI)

Slow-release carbohydrates and low-GI foods provide satiety and keep hunger at bay.

Diet history

While researching foods for persons with diabetes at the University of Toronto in the 1980s, Dr David Jenkins observed the speed at which foods were broken down by the body into glucose, the body's source of energy. His team devised the glycaemic index (GI) to measure the blood glucose raising potential of simple and complex carbohydrates. Many low-GI foods turned out to be whole or mixed grains, legumes, low-fat dairy, and some fruits and vegetables – findings that matched decade-old recommendations by nutritionists and doctors the world over.

How does it work?

In equivalent quantities, the complex carbohydrates in white bread elevate blood glucose levels more than the simple carbohydrates in ice cream, despite its sugar content. GI values rate carbs by their influence on blood glucose levels (quick versus slow release). The speed at which a given food is digested is measured by its GI against glucose, which scores 100. Most high-GI foods contain white flour and are heavily processed.

The diet is based on foods that slowly release sugar into the bloodstream for a steady supply of energy. This realization has changed traditional ideas about carbohydrates, their relationship to blood glucose and managing diabetes. The research can be applied to weight loss as high-GI foods cause hunger to return quickly.

treats

Primarily fruits. Also, baked items made with whole grains or nuts.

see also
good-carb low-carb 62

sample menu

Low-GI foods help prevent the

	saturday	sunday	monday	tuesday
morning	traditional porridge, honey, seeds and nuts	fruit yogurt	scrambled eggs on rye bread	wholewheat toast with peanut butter, low-fat milk
mid-morning	2 plums	1 apple or a handful of raspberries	½ a grapefuit	2 plums
lunch	tuna and bean salad	avocado and chicken salad	grilled pork chop, tomato, and spinach	grilled chicken breast, salad tuna and bean salad
mid-afternoon	10 grapes	1 orange or pear	10 grapes	1 orange or pear
supper	baked chicken breast and vegetables	baked cod, green beans, carrots and rice	baked trout with almonds, tomato, broccoli	avocado and ham salad
drinks	tea, decaf coffee, herbal teas, water	tea, decaf coffee, herbal teas, water	tea, decaf coffee, herbal teas, water	tea, decaf coffee, herbal teas, water

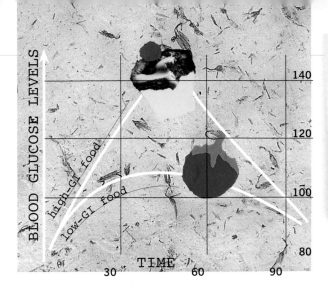

Graph: BLOOD GLUCOSE LEVELS (y-axis: 80, 100, 120, 140) vs TIME (x-axis: 30, 60, 90). Curves labelled high-GI food, low-GI food.

weigh this up...

- Glycaemic index is the measure of the type of carbohydrate in your food and ranges from low (multigrain bread) to high (white bread). The "glycaemic load" is a food's GI multiplied by its dietary carbohydrate content. Low-GI foods generally break down slowly, helping to give you a steady energy release and better balanced blood sugar levels.

Low-GI foods form the core of the diet because digested more slowly they leave you feeling fuller, for longer. Highly processed, sugary foods cause blood sugar levels to leap and the pancreas to release insulin.
As the sudden energy boost drops, hunger kicks in. With plenty of glucose in the blood, your body uses it over stored fat. So to lose weight, keep insulin levels low.

Some variations of the diet use food lists with high, medium or low GI ratings (55 or less is considered low). Other versions group foods into three categories: red (avoid if you want to lose weight), yellow (eat occasionally) and green (eat liberally).

Pros and cons
Medically and nutritionally sound, the GI Diet is also varied. Clinically proven benefits include lower blood glucose and insulin levels (ideal for diabetics). GI values have been identified for many foods but not for meals or food combinations due to the unlimited variations.

Is it for you?
The GI Diet helps reduce the risk of heart disease, stroke, type 2 diabetes, and colon and prostate cancer. The books and websites available make this programme a possible lifelong solution. You may need to carry a GI chart while you familiarize yourself with low- and high-GI foods. Home and restaurant dining GI-style is reasonably easy.

Availability
All of the foods in this diet can be readily purchased from any general food shop or supermarket.

Lifestyle changes
Physical activity is recommended.

forbidden foods

- certain meats and poultry
- certain vegetables
- some starches and baked foods
- whole milk
- alcohol
- sweets

hunger pangs that result from low blood sugar levels.

wednesday	thursday	friday
wholegrain cereal, wholewheat toast	wholegrain cereal, wholewheat toast	wholewheat toast with peanut butter
1 apple or a handful of raspberries	unsweetened apple sauce	2 plums
turkey salad sandwich	poached egg, wholewheat muffin	grilled chicken breast, salad
10 grapes	1 orange or pear	10 grapes
steak with guacamole	chargrilled beef with mushrooms	avocado and ham salad
tea, decaf coffee, herbal teas, water	tea, decaf coffee, herbal teas, water	tea, decaf coffee, herbal teas, water

Resources
www.gidiet.com

Brand-Miller, J, Foster-Powell, K., McMillan-Price, J. *The Low GI Diet Revolution* (2004, Marlowe and Co.)

Gallop, R. *Living the GI Diet* (2004, Workman Publishing Co.)

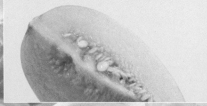

LONG-TERM PLAN

FLEXIBILITY

FAMILY FRIENDLY

COST

STRENGTH OF SCIENCE

LA SHAPE DIET

Ideal for a modern, fast-paced lifestyle and a relatively new arrival on the diet scene, this plan uses body shape and a personalised eating plan to determine specific protein requirements.

Diet history
This diet was developed by David Heber, founder of the UCLA Center for Human Nutrition, chairman of the Scientific and Medical Advisory Board of Herbalife International (a global distributor of nutritional supplements) and author of *What Color is Your Diet?* (2003).

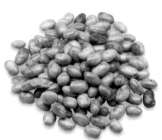

How does it work?
According to the LA Shape Diet, body shape and identifying differences in body fat distribution are key to determining an individual's ideal diet. Upper-body fat (apple-shape) cells and lower-body fat (pear-shape) cells serve different purposes and their distribution influences the success/failure of any weight-loss effort. A dietary intake of protein based on body shape and lean body mass can then be recommended to reduce hunger pangs.

This low-carbohydrate, low-fat, high-protein plan offers lifestyle strategies and additional dietary recommendations such as eating healthy carbohydrates, colourful fruits and vegetables and good fats to reduce and control hunger, plus recipes for high-protein "empowering shakes". These meal replacements are made from soya protein powder, protein powder (added to achieve the personal protein target),

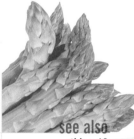

see also
atkins 42

sample menu
Shakes as meal replacements are temporary

	saturday One meal replacement (men)	sunday One meal replacement (men)	monday Two meal replacements	tuesday Two meal replacements
morning	Blueberry-Soya Protein Shake (with added protein for personal protein prescription), 1 cup coffee or tea	7 egg whites, chives, herbs, 180g spinach, 1 slice wholewheat toast, 1 cup coffee	Pumpkin-Banana Shake	Strawberry-Kiwi Shake
lunch	seafood salad (water-packed tuna, imitation crabmeat, tomatoes, celery, parsley, and green onion), LA Shape Green Goddess dressing, 1 slice wholegrain bread	Pineapple-Orange-Coconut Shake	Chocolate-Raspberry Shake	Chai Tea-Latte Shake
dinner	high-protein bar, banana	55g soya nuts, 1 orange	30g roasted soy nuts	½ protein bar
snacks	chicken and turkey meatloaf, steamed broccoli and carrots, 120g brown rice, baked cinnamon apple	prawn and vegetable kebabs, 2 tbsp barbecue sauce, vegetable salad	quick chicken soup, tossed green salad, LA Shape Green Goddess Dressing	Baja seafood cocktail, tossed green salad, LA Shape Green Goddess Dressing

240ml of soya or fat-free milk, 220g of fresh or frozen fruit and ice cubes. Meals consist of 80–120g of chicken, fish or turkey, 400g of steamed vegetables, 300g of salad with rice vinegar or wine vinegar and a fruit for dessert.

Pros and cons

Customized to meet individual needs, the plan addresses body fat percentage, not pounds shed, and includes lean meat, fruit, vegetables and behavioural strategies. The

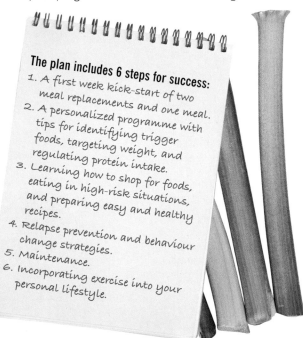

The plan includes 6 steps for success:

1. A first week kick-start of two meal replacements and one meal.
2. A personalized programme with tips for identifying trigger foods, targeting weight, and regulating protein intake.
3. Learning how to shop for foods, eating in high-risk situations, and preparing easy and healthy recipes.
4. Relapse prevention and behaviour change strategies.
5. Maintenance.
6. Incorporating exercise into your personal lifestyle.

daily dependence on shakes, however, may not allow for the integration of the skills necessary to manage weight successfully following three meals a day. Transfering or adding this to a regular food intake over the long term may contribute to excessive calorie intake. The focus on fresh foods requires regular shopping.

Is it for you?

The LA Shape Diet may appeal to healthy, active individuals who prefer a structured plan and enjoy fruit shakes. Those who wish to integrate three meals into their daily schedule may find it more challenging. Some dieters may not tolerate the emphasis placed on fruit and dietary supplements.

Availability

All of the foods included in this diet are readily available from any general supermarket or health food store.

Lifestyle changes

Goal setting, stress reduction, relapse prevention, social support, daily exercise, vitamin and mineral supplements, and self-monitoring are recommended as part of the plan.

forbidden foods

- fatty red meats
- butter
- cheese
- nuts
- pizza
- creamy salad dressing
- mayonnaise
- soft drinks
- fruit juice
- rice
- beans
- ice cream
- alcohol (including beer)

treats

PICK FROM:

- fish
- lean meats
- fresh fruit
- fruit shakes
- vegetables

and need to be replaced with healthy eating skills.

wednesday Two meal replacements	thursday One meal replacement (women)	friday One meal replacement (women)
Banana-Walnut Shake	Blueberry-Soya Protein Shake (with added protein for personal protein prescription)	7 egg whites, onion, chives, herbs, 1 slice wholewheat toast, cantaloupe
Pineapple-Orange-Coconut Shake	seafood salad (water-packed tuna, imitation crabmeat, tomatoes, celery, parsley and green onion), LA Shape Green Goddess dressing	Banana Shake
100g fat-free cottage cheese, 70g fresh fruit	1 banana or 1 orange	140g fresh or frozen blackberries or blueberries
chicken and vegetable kebabs, 2 tbsp barbecue sauce, vegetable salad	chicken and turkey meatloaf, steamed broccoli and carrots, baked cinnamon apple	soya chilli, salad of mixed field greens, LA Shape Green Goddess dressing, apple

Resources

www.lashapediet.com

www.chasefreedom.com/la_shape

Heber, D. *The New LA Shape Diet: The 14-Day Total Weight Loss Plan* (2004, Regan Books)

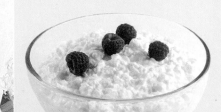

LONG-TERM PLAN

FLEXIBILITY

FAMILY FRIENDLY

COST

STRENGTH OF SCIENCE

NEANDERTHIN DIET

A low-carbohydrate plan based on the diet of paleolithic hunter-gatherers.

Diet history
The diet was developed by Ray Audette, for himself, in an effort to offset the effects of his diabetes and arthritis.

How does it work?
The assumption behind the plan is that the prehistoric diet is better than the modern diet. The rationale is that our modern diet is rooted in agriculture, the Industrial Revolution and technology, and largely responsible for many of today's health problems, including obesity. The Neanderthin Diet is supposedly designed to prevent obesity, which is considered an immune-system response to a diet that is the result of modern technology.

This "prehistoric diet" plan is based on meat, vegetables, fruit, nuts and berries. It is purported to be a healthy and effective way to lose weight. This is based on the idea that to eat more efficiently for our bodies, we should follow a diet similar to that eaten before the development of agriculture and technology.

The criteria for determining if a food is appropriate is basically, "Could I eat this if I were naked with a sharp stick on the savanna?"

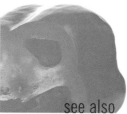

see also
atkins 42
scarsdale 60
raw food 174

sample menu
An easy planning guide: if you can't hunt or

	saturday	sunday	monday	tuesday	
morning	beef jerky, apple, almond butter, peppermint tea	pork spare ribs, scrambled eggs, salsa, Earl Grey tea	bacon, eggs, grapefruit juice	pork chops, eggs, canteloupe	
lunch	grilled halibut, artichoke, mushrooms and onions, watermelon, juice	baked chicken, steamed cauliflower, wild greens salad, Perrier water	chilli, tossed salad, steamed broccoli, iced tea	baked chicken, steamed marrow, sliced cucumber, mineral water	
supper	chicken soup, spinach salad with cucumber, tomato and avocado, iced green tea	green chilli stew, celery and carrot sticks, pineapple slices, tea	pork spare ribs, wild greens salad, steamed cauliflower, herbal tea	minced beef with pasta, steamed cauliflower, red pepper slices, iced tea	
snack 1	pork scratchings, papaya	hazelnuts, plum	almonds, apple	nut milk, melon	
snack 2	fruit ice	peach and pear salad	beef jerky	pecans	

weigh this up...

The diet has "Ten Commandments" that list five groups of allowed foods and five groups of foods to avoid.

- Do eat meat and fish, fruit, vegetables, nuts and seeds, berries.
- Do not eat grains (including maize and wheat), beans (including peanuts and soya), potatoes and other starchy vegetables, dairy products (including butter), sugar (including corn sweeteners).

This diet promotes "natural eating", defined as the absence of technology. According to the book, humans are genetically adapted to the paleolithic diet as a result of evolutionary selection.

However, this assumes that we have not continued evolving, that all the changes brought through agriculture, the Industrial Revolution, or technology offer no benefits to human nutrition, and must be rejected.

This is a low-carbohydrate, high-protein and high-fat diet. The paleolithic lifestyle is based on a type of physical activity and environment that are not common today (we no longer run naked in the savanna throughout the day hunting for food).

Pros and cons

The plan emphasizes eating foods in as natural a state as possible. Many of the meat and fish recommended on the plan (such as venison, elk, buffalo, moose, octopus, seal and eel) or nuts (such as acorns or hickory) are not readily available and unusual to many. Although it is generally desirable to limit consumption of refined foods, some of the food restrictions are unnecessary, for example wholewheat, corn, rye, beans, yams, milk and cheese can be part of a healthy diet. The emphasis on meats (some have a high saturated fat content), given today's relatively sedentary lifestyle, may increase the risk for some chronic diseases.

Is it for you?

This plan will appeal to those who like meat and vegetables, and can easily forgo grains. Many of the foods are wild game. It may be inappropriate or medically unsound for individuals with special medical conditions. It should not be started without medical supervision.

Availability

Most of the foods can be bought in a general food shop but some may need to be obtained from specialist suppliers.

Lifestyle changes

Increase physical activity and drink a lot of fresh water. Trying to follow this diet would likely require a big change in food acquisition patterns.

pick it, don't eat it.

wednesday	thursday	friday
rare rib-eye steak, pear, green tea	venison sausage patties, vegetable juice	omelette, orange juice
boiled prawns, steamed asparagus, carrots, peppermint tea	rabbit stew with tomatoes, celery, red peppers, fennel, shallots, leeks, hot cider	salad with tuna, wild greens, avocado, celery and cucumber slices, water
hamburger, avocado slices, tossed salad, steamed spinach, hot tea	baked chicken, steamed broccoli, sliced tomatoes, iced tea	chilli, red pepper slices, carrot sticks, iced tea
filberts, banana	sliced vegatables	walnuts, orange
beef jerky	dried fruits and nuts	oysters with lemon

Resources

www.beyondveg.com

www.lowcarb.ca/atkins-diet-and-low-carb-plans/neanderthin-diet.html

Audette, R. *Neanderthin* (1999, St. Martin's Press)

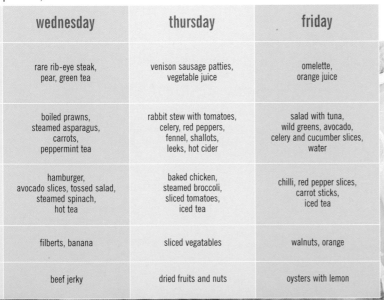

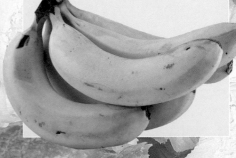

Note: Juices should be fresh or freshly squeezed. Recipes are included in the book *Neanderthin*.

THE NEW SUGAR BUSTERS!

A meal plan to make a permanent lifestyle change by eliminating high glycaemic index foods and beverages.

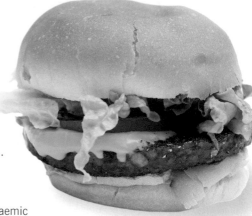

Tofu burger with fat-free cheese.

Diet history
Sugar Busters! Cut Sugar to Trim Fat was published in 1995. The authors of the book include H. Leighton Steward, a former CEO; Morrison C. Bethea, MD, a cardiothoracic surgeon; Samuel S. Andrews, MD, an endocrinologist; and Luis A. Balart, MD, a gastroenterologist. A revised and updated edition of the book, *The New Sugar Busters! Cut Sugar to Trim Fat* was more recently released.

How does it work?
The diet's claim is that by consuming the correct carbohydrates, which are those lower on the glycaemic index, insulin resistance in individuals can be reduced. The allowed carbohydrates are those that result in low insulin production. The rationale is that insulin causes the body to convert and store excess sugar and fat as fat. (But excess calories, whether from carbohydrates, fat or protein, are stored as fat.)

Late-night snacking is not allowed because it is supposed to increase insulin levels and encourage cholesterol production. From a behaviour modification standpoint it is good to avoid the habit of

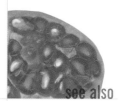

see also
good-carb low-carb 62
south beach 64

LONG-TERM PLAN

FLEXIBILITY

FAMILY FRIENDLY

COST
●

STRENGTH OF SCIENCE

sample menu
This menu emphasizes selecting foods that are

	saturday	sunday	monday	tuesday
morning	scrambled eggs (in rapeseed oil), grapefruit, skimmed milk	wholewheat pancake, fresh blackberries, back bacon, decaf coffee	wholegrain porridge, small orange, skimmed milk	omelette with onion, mushroom and tomato, grapes, hot green tea (plain)
lunch	vegetable soup, wholegrain bread, dark green salad with walnuts and strawberries, water	split pea soup, peanut butter and no-added-sugar jam sandwich, skimmed milk	spinach salad with mandarin oranges, vegetable barley soup, skimmed milk	tuna salad (in water) on cos lettuce, wholegrain crackers, celery sticks, skimmed milk
supper	lean pork loin, steamed spinach, wholegrain rice pilaf with flaked almonds, skimmed milk	grilled white fish, brown basmati rice, steamed courgettes, wholewheat bread, water	grilled salmon, baked sweet potato, steamed asparagus, water	lean steak, steamed green beans, apricot slices, wholewheat dinner roll, water
snack 1	soya nuts (handful)	pumpkin seeds (handful)	hard-boiled egg	½ avocado with lemon juice
snack 2	nectarine	pomegranate	no-added-sugar ice cream	kiwi fruit

eating snacks late at night, since these snacks are frequently high in calories. Insulin levels would not be significantly increased if the snack was a serving of lean meat, or other high-protein food, and water.

The diet claims that most of the fat on our bodies comes from sugar and not fat. However, excess body fat is due to the consumption of too many calories, regardless of the food source. When foods are limited or not allowed, as with Sugar Busters!, a decrease in calories consumed will most likely occur. This will lead to a decrease in body fat, which may help decrease insulin resistance. Scientific evidence supports the idea that a decrease in overall daily calorie intake promotes weight loss and that maintaining a healthy body weight may help in the prevention of insulin resistance and type 2 diabetes.

Pros and cons

Choosing foods high in fibre, low in total and saturated trans fats, and reducing portion sizes, are encouraged. Sugar Busters! now has a shopper's guide, a cookery book and a book for kids.

But some healthy foods and all refined sugars are avoided and the glycaemic load of meals is not calculated – only the glycaemic index of individual foods and drinks is considered. Permanently avoiding foods and drinks that are not allowed may be unrealistic and even frustrating for some.

Dining out may be challenging because it is necessary to know the glycaemic index of the foods and drinks. Also, since this is a permanent lifestyle change, avoiding "unacceptable" foods forever may be difficult.

Is it for you?

Since Sugar Busters is promoted as a lifestyle – not a diet – it may suit individuals who want to make permanent changes in their eating habits. It may also suit those who have diabetes, are insulin resistant, or trying to lose weight.

The foods in this meal plan are healthy and are appropriate for nearly everyone if the menus are nutritionally balanced, which may be difficult to do without guidance.

Availability

Most of the foods in this diet are available from your local grocery shop or a large supermarket.

Lifestyle changes

Physical activity is encouraged.

forbidden foods

- beetroot
- sweetcorn
- red or white potatoes
- bananas (ripe)
- pineapples
- raisins
- large amounts of watermelon
- fried chicken
- baked beans
- regular colas

healthy tips

- Drink skimmed or soya milk with meals or snacks to increase calcium intake.
- Drink six to eight glasses of water daily.

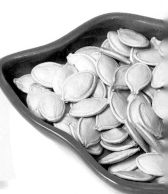

low glycaemic index.

	wednesday	thursday	friday
	wholegrain cereal with skimmed milk, fresh peach slices, decaf coffee	poached egg, 1 slice wholewheat toast, freshly squeezed orange juice	high-fibre, wholegrain cereal with skimmed milk, fresh raspberries, hot green tea (plain)
	tofu burger with fat-free cheese, onion, lettuce and tomato, tangerine, skimmed milk	wholewheat pitta with hummus, tabbouleh, apple slices, skimmed milk	fruit plate with fat-free cottage cheese, cantaloupe and honeydew, black bean soup, water
	grilled chicken, steamed broccoli with red pepper, wild rice, water	grilled white fish, steamed cauliflower and carrots, mixed strawberry and blueberry cup, water	baked turkey breast, steamed sugar-snap peas, wholegrain couscous, skimmed milk
	celery sticks with peanut butter	plum	fat-free cheese stick
	plain, fat-free yogurt with blueberries	walnuts (handful)	fresh pear

Notes: 100% wholewheat or wholegrain breads and oatmeal should be used. Drink six to eight glasses of water daily.

Resources

www.sugarbusters.com/books_pyrimad.php

www.glycemicindex.com

Steward, H. L., Bethea, M., Andrews, S., Balart, L. *The New Sugar Busters! Cut Sugar To Trim Fat* (2003, Ballantine Books)

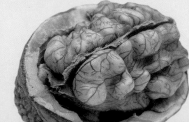

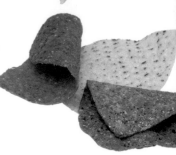

PRITIKIN DIET

Devised for maintaining a healthy heart and also for weight loss, this low-fat plan uses food exchange lists, exercise and stress management.

LONG-TERM PLAN

FLEXIBILITY

FAMILY FRIENDLY

COST
●

STRENGTH OF SCIENCE

Diet history
Based on personal health issues, the original diet was developed in the 1950s by Nathan Pritikin, founder of the Pritikin Longevity Center. Several books by Robert Pritikin, his son, have since advanced and promoted the diet. Although its popularity continues to fluctuate, the centre has been successful and is respected for its treatment and research.

How does it work?
Currently established as a lifetime plan for healthy living through diet, exercise and stress management, the Pritikin Diet was originally developed for the prevention and treatment of heart disease. Very low in fat, high in fibre and with a daily exercise component, the diet's popularity increased primarily as a result of the related weight loss.

  The plan is comprised of a total caloric breakdown of 10 per cent fats, 10–15 per cent proteins, and 75–80 per cent carbohydrates with daily amounts of at least 35 grams of fibre, less than 100 milligrams of cholesterol, and 600 milligrams of sodium. Food exchange lists are used and foods are categorized into "go, caution and stop".

Tortilla chips are allowed as a treat.

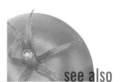

see also
dean ornish 48
volumetrics 108

sample menu
This low-fat diet was developed to prevent heart

	saturday	sunday	monday	tuesday
morning	50g shredded wheat, 100g blueberries, 1 glass skimmed milk	200g cooked oatmeal, 2 tbsp raisins, 1 glass skimmed milk	½ wholewheat bagel, ½ cantaloupe, 110g fat-free cream cheese	25g shredded wheat, ½ banana, 1 glass skimmed milk
snack 1	50g green pepper strips	240ml celery vegetable juice	120ml low-sodium vegetable juice	1 carrot
lunch	cos lettuce with 15g cooked turkey, grapefruit, lime and tomatillo salsa, baked cornmeal chips, 110g mango	240ml low-fat Mediterranean lentil soup, 10 wholewheat crackers, 225ml pineapple	1 slice wholewheat bread, 105g salad with fat-free dressing, 110g dry curd cottage cheese, 1 pear	1 slice brown bread, 40g vegetarian baked beans, 110g steamed vegetables, apple
supper	200g wholewheat pasta, 80g prawns and cherry tomatoes, 100g spinach salad, 100g grapes	1 baked potato, 100g grilled scallops, 100g beetroot, 180g mange-tout, 100g salad, 1 tsp safflower oil, mango smoothie	100g wholewheat pasta, 75ml marinara sauce, 100g chicken strips, peach and orange juice spritzer (with 120ml juice)	100g grilled fish sticks, 1 baked potato, 2 tsp olive oil, 110g dry curd cottage cheese, 175g broccoli
snack 2	55g wholewheat pretzels, 1 celery stalk	280ml orange juice, cinnamon-flavoured rice cake	2 brown rice cakes, 100g cherry tomatoes	75g plain popcorn, 50g carrot and jicama sticks, 1 tbsp fat-free ranch dressing

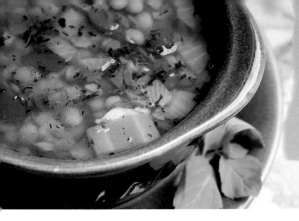

treats

PICK FROM:
- **yogurt parfait**
- **banana ice cream**
- **cheesecake**
- **apple date cake**
- **tortilla chips**
- **fruit syrup**

Low-fat Mediterranean lentil soup (left) is an ideal lunchtime meal.

forbidden foods
- **animal fats**
- **hydrogenated oils**
- **fatty meats**
- **coconut**
- **whole dairy products**
- **salt**
- **egg yolks**
- **caffeinated drinks**

The fast-track weight-loss plan is of 1,000 calories (for women) and 1,200 calories (for men), with complex, high-fibre carbohydrates encouraged. The newer plan also focuses on foods that are not calorie dense.

Pros and cons
This holistic approach to dieting is good for weight reduction and protects the heart. Its emphasis on fruits, vegetables and wholegrain foods will suit vegetarians. Encouraged as a lifelong lifestyle commitment, this restrictive, low-fat, high-fibre plan requires planning and may be difficult to integrate within a daily routine. The fact is adequate amounts of calcium are difficult to obtain without resorting to fortified foods and must be carefully considered if following the diet over the long term.

Is it for you?
This is not a diet designed for rapid weight loss but more of a lifestyle plan for those interested in a holistic disease but is also used for weight loss.

approach to promoting heart health in addition to weight loss.

This very low-fat diet includes a very restrictive "fast-track" weight-loss plan that only allows 1,000 calories (for women) and 1,200 calories (for men). It is therefore especially important that people with medical conditions consult a doctor beforehand.

Availability
The foods in the diet can be purchased in any supermarket but shopping will involve careful label reading and product comparison.

Lifestyle changes
Exercise and stress management are integral to the plan.

wednesday	thursday	friday
100g cooked porridge, 2 tbsp raisins, 1 glass skimmed milk	½ wholewheat bagel, 2 tbsp raisins, 110g fat-free cream cheese	55g wholewheat cereal flakes, ½ banana, 1 glass skimmed milk
110g orange sections	1 glass low-sodium tomato juice	120ml low-sodium tomato juice
½ pitta bread, 200g spinach, 2 tbsp almonds, 300g strawberries, 2 tbsp fat-free dressing, 100g red pepper sticks	240ml fat-free Santa Fe vegetarian soup, 100g salad, 1 kiwi fruit	1 pitta, 200g Italian-style vegetables, 120ml low-fat marinara sauce, 200g green salad, 220g honeydew
½ pitta bread, 100g baked chicken, 80ml salsa, 110g fruit cocktail, 110g low-fat yogurt	1 baked potato, 200g mixed vegetable salad, 100g grilled salmon, peach smoothie with 1 peach and 1 glass skimmed milk	110g brown rice, 175g broccoli and cauliflower medley, 100g baked flounder, cinnamon apple rings
1 baked potato, 100g chopped broccoli	75g plain popcorn, 100g red pepper strips	1 multigrain rice cake, 1 carrot

Resources
www.pritikin.com

www.webmd.com/content/pages/7/3220_282.htm

Pritikin, R. *The Pritikin Principle* (2000, Time Life Books)

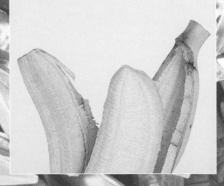

LONG-TERM PLAN

FLEXIBILITY

FAMILY FRIENDLY
●

COST
●●

STRENGTH OF SCIENCE

SCARSDALE DIET

This restrictive two-week diet cuts out fats, most dairy products, carbs, fruit juice, alcohol, desserts and deli meat.

Diet history
Developed by Dr Herman Tarnower, the Scarsdale Diet was one of the first popular low-carbohydrate diets but has since been eclipsed by trendier equivalents.

How does it work?
This low-calorie, high-protein, low-carbohydrate plan consists of a 1,000-calorie daily allowance based around the three standard mealtimes (breakfast, lunch and dinner). The Scarsdale emphasis is on lean meat and poultry without the skin, vegetables and fruit. Drinking plenty of water or fluids, such as diet, is also encouraged. After two weeks of strict dieting, individuals are encouraged to switch over to the Keep Trim Program which includes an extended "allowed" foods list.

The initial two weeks of the plan are ultra low in calories and very strict, forbidding any kinds of substitutes and alcohol. The claim is that this regime produces ketones but no more than desirable.

The Scarsdale Diet's Keep Trim component is also restrictive and allows only two slices of "protein" or wholewheat bread per day.

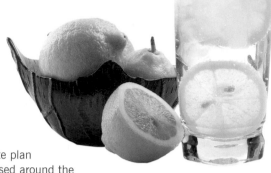

It is important to drink lots of water when following high-protein diets.

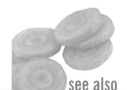

see also
atkins 42
south beach 64

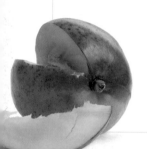

sample menu
Meal planning is easy – the diet is based on

	saturday	sunday	monday	tuesday
morning	½ grapefruit, 1 slice high-protein bread, tea	½ grapefruit, 1 slice wholewheat bread, coffee	½ grapefruit, 1 slice wholewheat bread, coffee	½ grapefruit, 1 slice high-protein bread, tea
lunch	100g low-fat cottage cheese, sliced fruit, 6 pecans, diet cola	lean grilled chicken breast, mixed vegetables (tomatoes, carrots, cabbage and broccoli), melon, tea	lean turkey and beef, sliced tomatoes, diet cola	large fruit salad, diet cola
supper	roast chicken, sliced tomatoes, lettuce, grapefruit, coffee	grilled steak, steamed Brussels sprouts, mixed salad (cucumber, tomato and lettuce), tea	grilled cod, carrot and cucumber salad, 1 slice high-protein bread, berries, coffee	grilled lean hamburger, cucumber, tomato and celery salad, steamed, Brussels sprouts, tea
snack 1	diet cola	water, celery	coffee	tea, celery
snack 2	coffee, carrots	tea	tea, carrots	diet cola

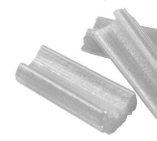

It prohibits sugar, potatoes, spaghetti, peanut butter, sweets, desserts, foods containing flour, cream, whole milk, fatty meats, dressings and fats. Special items, such as high-protein bread, must be purchased or homemade. Carrots, celery, fruit and sugar-free jellies are allowed.

Pros and cons

To its credit, this highly structured programme includes lean meat, fruit and vegetables but the downsides include its ultra-low calorie content, the carbohydrate intake restriction and limited meal options, which some dieters may find quite repetitive in the long run. As with other diets which promise rapid weight loss, the pounds will come back on once you resume your normal eating habits. Note that some of the data in the book (such as the weight-to-height table) are now out of date.

Is it for you?

The Scarsdale Diet is likely to attract those who like eating meat and want a drastic, short-term plan for rapid weight loss. Anyone with diabetes, kidney disease and other health complications or who is pregnant should avoid this and other high-protein, low-calorie diets. The programme is aimed at healthy people but do consult your doctor first.

Availability

All of the foods in this diet are readily available and can be bought from any general food shop or supermarket.

healthy tips

- You are only allowed to snack on carrots, celery, coffee, tea, soda water or diet sodas between meals.
- Low-fat cottage cheese with 1 tbsp low-fat sour cream, fruit and nuts can substitute any lunch.

Lifestyle changes

Although exercise is not part of the plan, the book does provide an exercise calorie chart. Daily weighing is recommended and dieters are encouraged to follow the regime whenever they are four pounds heavier than their desired weight.

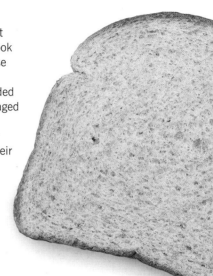

lean meat and vegetables.

wednesday	thursday	friday	Resources
½ grapefruit, 1 slice high-protein bread, tea	½ grapefruit, 1 slice wholewheat bread, coffee	½ grapefruit, 1 slice high-protein bread, tea	lowcarblisa.tripod.com
tuna dressed with vinegar, melon, water	2 hard-boiled eggs, lettuce, tomato, celery, and cucumber salad, water	lean chicken and turkey, grilled tomatoes, diet cola	thescarsdalemedicaldiet/id18.html www.skinnyondiets.com/ TheCompleteScarsdaleMedical Diet.html
lean grilled lamb, lettuce, cucumber and tomato salad, coffee	roast pork fillets, spinach and green pepper salad, steamed green beans, tea	grilled prawns, grilled mushrooms, green salad, 1 slice high-protein bread, tea	Tarnower, H. and Sinclair-Baker, S. *The Complete Scarsdale Medical Diet Plus Dr. Tarnower's Lifetime Keep-Slim Program* (1978, Bantam Books)
diet cola	coffee	tea, celery	
coffee	water, carrots	diet cola	

Note: There are recipes available in the book.

LONG-TERM PLAN
●●●

FLEXIBILITY
●●

FAMILY FRIENDLY
●●

COST
●

STRENGTH OF SCIENCE
●●

SECRETS OF GOOD-CARB LOW-CARB LIVING

This diet provides an overview of how to live on a healthy, low-carbohydrate diet by incorporating low-carbohydrate eating into an overall healthy lifestyle.

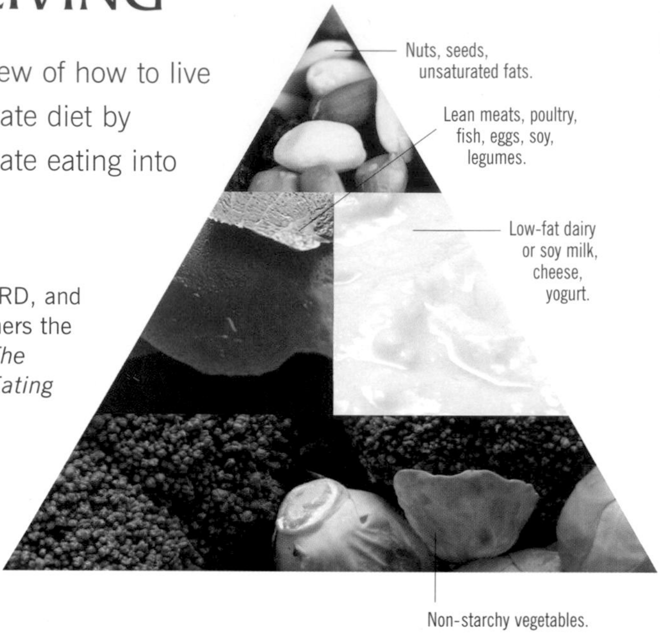

Diet history
Created by Sandra Woodruff, MS, RD, and published in 2004, this book furthers the ideas discussed her earlier book, *The Good Carb Cookbook: Secrets of Eating Low on the Glycemic Index.*

How does it work?
This programme offers two phases. The optional "Low-Carb Quick-Start Program" encourages a kick-start to weight loss by allowing mostly non-starchy vegetables, lean protein (including meat, poultry, fish, eggs, soya and legumes), low-fat dairy or soya products, and heart-healthy fats from nuts, seeds and unsaturated fats. This is adequate in nutrients and does not generate ketones, unlike some other low-carbohydrate diets.

After the initial phase, the "Good-Carb Life Plan" is recommended

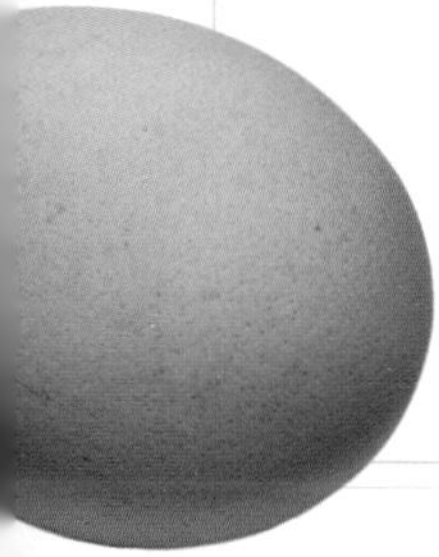

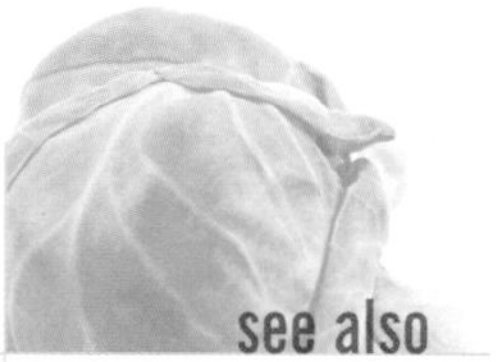

Nuts, seeds, unsaturated fats.

Lean meats, poultry, fish, eggs, soy, legumes.

Low-fat dairy or soy milk, cheese, yogurt.

Non-starchy vegetables.

see also
glycaemic index 50
south beach 64

sample menu

The menu, if well planned, will contain the

	saturday	sunday	monday	tuesday
morning	scrambled eggs, vegetarian sausage patty, skimmed milk	low-fat, sugar-free flavoured yogurt, hard-boiled egg	vegetable omelette, vegetarian sausage link	scrambled eggs with ham and spinach, skimmed milk
lunch	mushroom caps with pizza topping, green salad with light vinaigrette dressing	meat and cheese lettuce wraps, broth-based soup	lentil soup with meat, vegetable lettuce wraps	grilled chicken salad with nuts and low-fat cheese, low-sodium bean soup
supper	roast beef, cooked cauliflower	grilled chicken and vegetables, cooked beans	vegetable lasagne, green salad with light vinaigrette and low-fat crumbled cheese	grilled fish, cooked green beans, tossed salad with light vinaigrette dressing
snack	meat and cheese wrapped in lettuce	mixed nuts	low-fat, sugar-free flavoured milk	low-fat, sugar-free flavoured yogurt

for making reduced-carbohydrate living a reality for life. This lifetime phase includes fruit and whole grains as the main source of carbohydrates and focuses on eliminating refined carbohydrates, such as white sugar and flour. The author explains how to use the glycaemic index and glycaemic load to help make healthy food choices. Exercise is also highly encouraged as the other necessary component for weight loss.

Recent research has shown that some types of low-carbohydrate diets can be successful for short-term weight loss. Reducing the amount of carbohydrate in the diet can help to prevent long-term weight gain, overeating, cardiovascular disease, diabetes, cancer and polycystic ovarian syndrome.

Pros and cons

This book is a comprehensive guide for anyone wishing to live a reduced-carbohydrate lifestyle in the long term. The "Good-Carb Plan for Life" teaches how to include the best type of carbohydrates and whole grains in the right proportions. This is a great plan for post-Atkins followers who want to find a way to include some carbohydrates in their diet. It is easy to read and full of tips. The book includes about 100 recipes.

> **weigh this up...**
> • Permitted foods for low-carb quick-start include lean meat, skinless poultry, seafood, tofu, vegetarian meat substitutes, legumes, low-fat dairy products, non-starchy vegetables, salad vegetables, heart-healthy fats (from nuts, seeds, avocados, olive oil and rapeseed oil), trans fat-free margarine and low-sugar salad dressings.

The disadvantage is that following the "Low-Carb Quick-Start Program" means spending extra time planning and preparing foods because it differs from the typical British high-carbohydrate diet. However, this is no different from many other healthy eating plans.

Is it for you?

This programme will appeal to those who like a reduced-carbohydrate diet. Some research suggests that a higher (but not extremely high) protein diet is appropriate for people as they age and for those who wish to increase their muscle tissue.

Medical supervision is very important for people who are on diabetes or blood pressure medication and are trying a reduced-carbohydrate diet for the first time. Those who have kidney or liver disease should consult their doctor before starting a high-protein diet.

Availability

Most of the foods in this diet are available from your local supermarket.

Lifestyle changes

As well as the change in eating habits, one hour of daily exercise is highly recommended.

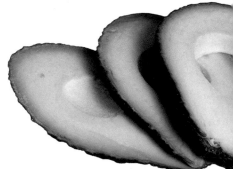

nutrients needed to support a healthy diet.

wednesday	thursday	friday
scrambled eggs substitute with low-fat cheese and herbs, vegetarian sausage patty, tomato juice	omelette with seasoned chicken, slice of avocado, tomato juice	sugar-free powdered nutrition shake, hard-boiled egg
meat chilli, green salad with light dressing	minced beef lettuce wraps, vegetable soup	Cobb salad, bean soup
grilled chicken, Brussels sprouts, green salad with light dressing	grilled pork loin, steamed vegetables, spinach salad	white fish with sautéed vegetables, tomato slices
celery stalk and peanut butter	tuna salad on lettuce leaves	almonds

Resources

www.ediets.com/glee/article.cfm/cmi_2426010/cid_35/code_30171

Woodruff, S. *Secrets of Good-Carb Low-Carb Living* (2004, Avery)

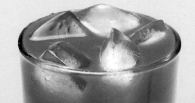

LONG-TERM PLAN

FLEXIBILITY

FAMILY FRIENDLY

COST

STRENGTH OF SCIENCE

SOUTH BEACH DIET

This high-protein plan initially restricts carbohydrates before re-introducing them in limited amounts.

Diet history
Developed by A. Agatston, MD, this plan was on the *New York Times* bestseller list and is a more liberal variation of the high-protein, low-carbohydrate plan.

How does it work?
The three-phase plan initially cuts down on "right" or "good" carbohydrates, then gradually re-introduces some back into the diet. Sources of protein include fish, chicken, turkey, lean veal, pork, beef, lamb, yogurt and low-fat cheeses; fats from nuts, olive, rapeseed and peanut oil; and snacks on the go. Serving sizes are specified with an emphasis on whole grains and low glycaemic index foods.

During the two weeks of Phase 1, lean meats, chicken, egg, egg substitutes, fish and olive oil are allowed. The major sources of carbohydrates are vegetables, salads, nuts and some low-fat milk.

Phase 2 re-introduces lower glycaemic index carbohydrate foods in limited amounts. This phase lasts for two weeks or until the desired weight is lost. Overindulging means returning to phase 1 for a week.

Fruits are recommended with lunch or dinner but not breakfast. Wholegrain bread, sweet potatoes or brown or wild rice replace white bread, white potatoes and white rice. Modest portions of rice or

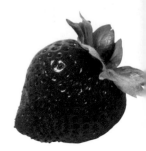

Prawns are a source of high-quality protein and are low in calories.

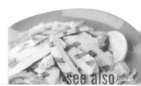

see also
atkins 42
scarsdale 60

sample menu
If you over-indulge, simply return to Phase 1 for

	saturday	sunday	monday	tuesday
morning	vegetable quiche cup with spinach, tomato juice, decaf coffee with skimmed milk	2-egg omelette with cheese, tomato juice, decaf coffee with skimmed milk	2 poached eggs, back bacon, vegetable juice, decaf coffee with skimmed milk	2-egg omelette with asparagus, back bacon, tomato juice, decaf tea
snack 1	turkey roll-up, coriander mayo	hummus and celery sticks	low-fat mozzarella cheese stick	low-fat cheddar cheese stick
lunch	salad greens with grilled chicken, oil and vinegar dressing	salad greens with grilled beef strips, oil and vinegar dressing	salad greens with grilled chicken, oil and vinegar dressing	salad greens with tuna, oil and vinegar dressing
supper	grilled salmon, steamed asparagus and mushrooms, tossed greens with olive oil	grilled tilapia, steamed kale with bacon bits, roasted aubergine and peppers, rocket salad with vinegar	grilled cod, roasted mixed vegetables, tossed salad with olive oil	grilled pork fillet, grilled tomatoes and pepper strips, shredded cabbage
snack 2	plain cashews	plain brazil nuts	plain almonds	vanilla-flavoured low-fat ricotta cheese*
snack 3	sugar-free gelatine	lemon-flavoured low-fat ricotta cheese*	sugar-free jelly, cherry tomatoes	plain cashews

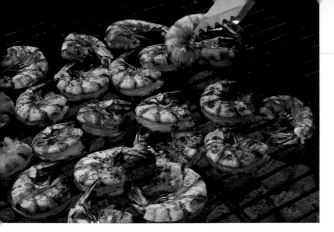

potatoes are allowed. Mashed steamed cauliflower replaces mashed potatoes. Sandwiches are replaced by fillings in lettuce-leaf wraps. Phase 3 is the lifelong weight maintenance stage where the consumption of some carbohydrates and fats is discouraged and an adherence to some basic rules is necessary.

This low-calorie, high-protein, low-carbohydrate plan allows healthy fats, high-fibre foods and selected carbohydrates in moderate amounts. The evidence suggests that moderate portions of carbohydrates, proteins and healthy fats facilitate weight management.

Pros and cons

The South Beach Diet is a variation on the carbohydrate-restricted diets which some people find quite challenging to follow. It is also likely to be low in calcium. Restrictive Phase 1 promotes quick weight loss, probably as the result of low caloric intake and related water loss. The long-term Phase 3 is often missing from similar diets.

Is it for you?

The South Beach Diet is likely to appeal to someone looking for quick initial weight loss, who likes some menu structure and limits on carbohydrates, but does not want to have to measure out or weigh food. Those who cannot live without potatoes, white bread, cereal, rice, pasta or corn should avoid it. Anyone with special health conditions should consult a physician or a registered dietician before trying the plan.

Availability

All the foods in this diet can be readily bought from any general foodstore or supermarket.

Lifestyle changes

Although the plan is not dependent on exercise, it does indicate that this would make the programme even more efficient.

forbidden foods

PHASE ONE:
- bread
- rice
- potatoes
- some vegetables
- pasta
- baked products
- beer

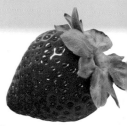

treats

PICK FROM:
- nuts
- some chocolate-flavoured desserts
- desserts made with low-fat ricotta cheese
- some types of berries
- sugar-free jelly

one week to get back on track.

wednesday	thursday	friday
2-egg omelette with broccoli, vegetable juice, back bacon, decaf coffee	frittata with ham and asparagus, tomato juice, decaf coffee with skimmed milk	2-egg omelette with peppers, back bacon, vegetable juice, decaf tea
rolled ham slice, celery sticks	low-fat cheddar cheese stick	sugar-free jelly
salad greens with turkey breast strips, oil and vinegar dressing	salad greens with grilled prawns, oil and vinegar dressing	1 grilled tomato stuffed with tuna salad
gazpacho, grilled mushroom caps, sautéed spinach, steamed julienne courgettes and butternut squash	grilled lean pork chop, grilled courgettes and butternut squash, steamed mange-tout	grilled turkey breast, steamed broccoli, mashed cauliflower, cucumber salad
plain pistachios	plain filberts	ricotta cheese, sugar-free chocolate syrup
sugar-free jelly, fat-free mozzarella stick	almond-flavoured low-fat ricotta cheese*	plain walnuts

Resources

www.southbeachdiet.com

www.lowcarb.ca/atkins-diet-and-low-carb-plans/south-beach-diet.html

Agatston, A. *The South Beach Diet* (2003, St. Martin's Press)

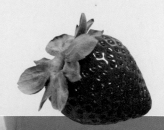

*Use extract for flavouring and sugar substitutes to sweeten, preferably derived from a complex sugar.

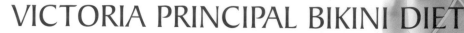

LONG-TERM PLAN

FLEXIBILITY

FAMILY FRIENDLY
●

COST
●

STRENGTH OF SCIENCE
●

VICTORIA PRINCIPAL BIKINI DIET

This "emergency" bikini-ready plan promises to help you lose 2–4kg in just seven days.

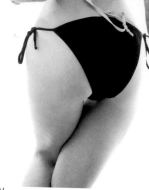

Diet history

Although the original diet was created by actress Victoria Principal and published in *The Diet Principal* (1987), there are other plans called the Bikini Diet. The celebrity status and fast weight-loss claims of her version, however, make it the most popular.

How does it work?

According to the Victoria Principal Bikini Diet, a 2–4kg (5–10lb) weight loss is guaranteed simply by following the set menu for one week. This "emergency" diet, however, should not be repeated more than once a year. Ultra low in calories and low in bulk (probably because of the small number of serving portions), this eating plan includes some fruit, vegetables and lean meats. Meals are to be strictly followed and no eating should take place after 8 p.m. Serving sizes are given so the actual measuring of food is not required. The consumption of many kinds of food is restricted either because of their caloric content or ingredient content (sodium and caffeine). It is recommended that you eat at home to avoid temptation and prevent a piling up of extra calories. Women are encouraged to take an additional calcium supplement to prevent the risk of osteoporosis. Ultimately, weight loss is possible because of the limitations imposed on the kinds of foods that are allowed and the serving sizes.

see also
scarsdale 60
ultrasimple 122

sample menu
The Bikini Diet should be followed exactly for

	saturday	sunday	monday	tuesday
morning	water, mixed melon salad, wholewheat toast, hot tea	water, prune juice, wholewheat crackers, decaf coffee	water, scrambled egg substitute, wholewheat toast, hot tea	water, prune juice, wholewheat crackers, decaf coffee
lunch	light tea, chicken salad with lettuce and cherry tomatoes, wholewheat crackers, lemonade	light tea, greens, tomato and tuna salad with balsamic vinegar, diet limeade	water, tossed greens salad (any vegetables but no tomatoes), turkey breast, hot tea	light tea, greens, tomato and tuna salad with balsamic vinegar, diet limeade
supper	water, grilled tilapia, sliced tomato, balsamic vinegar, celery sticks, decaf coffee	water, grilled chicken, steamed vegetables, wholewheat crackers, iced tea	water, steamed winter vegetable combination with any grated cheese, diet lemonade	water, consommé, steamed vegetables, chicken breast, skimmed milk
snack 1	light tea	water	water	light tea
snack 2	water	light tea	light tea	water

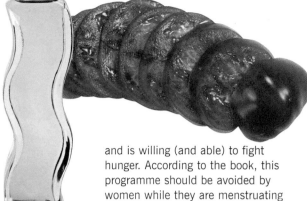

healthy tips

• To curb appetite levels, consume over eight glasses of water a day, remembering to drink one glass of water or light tea before each meal and another one straight after eating, with two additional glasses or cups between meals.

Pros and cons

This one-week diet presents the dieter with a detailed menu plan for the whole week, which makes it easy to follow. Each daily menu provides some variety, and useful tips are given for dining out.

Designed to be followed with precision, this calorie-restricted diet could leave you feeling hungry. Some weight loss occurs due to the low number of calories and not the foods per se, but most comes from loss of water and muscle – not fat.

Is it for you?

This diet is likely to appeal to someone who wants to kick-start noticeable weight loss using a structured plan, and is willing (and able) to fight hunger. According to the book, this programme should be avoided by women while they are menstruating and by anyone with medical conditions. Those not in good health should consult their doctor before starting the plan.

Availability

All of the foods recommended for this diet can be readily purchased from any general food shop or supermarket and do not require elaborate preparation methods of any kind.

Lifestyle changes

None. More permanent lifestyle changes are provided for the other diets featured in the book such as the 30-Day Diet and Diet for Life.

forbidden foods

• dairy products
• canned foods
• oil-based salad dressings
• sugar
• alcohol
• coffee and caffeine
• diet colas

free foods

• water
• teas

one week, with no substitutes.

wednesday	thursday	friday
water, tomato slices, wholewheat toast, low-calorie dressing, decaf coffee	water, scrambled egg substitute, wholewheat toast, decaf coffee	water, tomato slices, wholewheat toast, decaf coffee
water, chicken or turkey salad, wholewheat crackers, tea	light tea, mixed vegetables, skimmed milk	light tea, tossed salad with prawns, low-calorie Italian dressing, diet limeade
water, steamed mixed vegetables with grated Parmesan cheese, diet lemonade	water, grilled cod, wholewheat crackers, steamed summer squash, tea	water, steamed summer vegetable combination with grated romano cheese, hot tea
water	light tea	water
light tea	water	light tea

Resources

www.victoriaprincipal.com

diet.ivillage.com/plans/0,,8h95,00.html

Principal, V. *Living Principal* (2001, Villard)

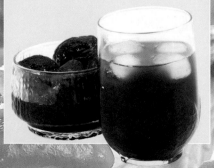

LONG-TERM PLAN

FLEXIBILITY

FAMILY FRIENDLY

COST

STRENGTH OF SCIENCE

ZONE DIET

This programme balances protein and carbohydrate ratios instead of calories as an approach to health and weight loss through food combinations that help you stay in the "zone".

Diet history

Born of his desire to avoid dying of a heart attack, the biochemist and nutrition scientist Barry Sears developed the Zone Diet and introduced it to the world in 1995. He is the author of several *New York Times* bestsellers and his many books include *Enter The Zone* (1995), *Zone-Perfect Meals in Minutes* (1997), *Zone Food Blocks* (1998), *The Zone: A Dietary Road Map* (1999), *The Age-Free Zone* (2000), *Mastering the Zone* (2001), *The Soy Zone* (2001), *The Omega Rx Zone* (2002), *Zone Perfect Cookbook* (2003), *What to Eat in the Zone* (2003), *A Week in the Zone* (2004), *The Top 100 Zone Foods* (2004), *Zone Meals in Seconds* (2004), *Zone Life Plan* (2005) and *The Anti-Inflammatory Zone* (2006). His books have sold more than five million copies and have been translated into 22 languages in 40 countries. Today he conducts research on the inflammatory process as president of the non-profit Inflammation Research Foundation in Massachusetts.

see also
south beach 64
mediterranean 160

sample menu

This diet's menus provide close to the recommended

	saturday	sunday	monday	tuesday
morning	1 scone, 1½ soya sausage patties, 30g cheese	egg whites, onions, mushrooms, spinach, 30g cheese, 140g fruit cocktail	breakfast quesadilla, 170g grapes	plain bagel, 80g smoked salmon, 3 tbsp light cream cheese
lunch	cheese omelette: 200g pasturised egg substitute, 30g cheese, olive oil spray, 120ml salsa	chicken salad with 4 tsp light mayonnaise in mini pitta pocket, ½ orange	1 slice bread, 55g ham, lettuce, tomato, 30g cheese, 100g yogurt	1 bowl chilli, 30g shredded cheese
supper	110g chicken, garlic, onions, peppers, mushrooms, spinach, 1 tbsp olive oil and vinegar dressing, 80g grapes	110g grilled pork loin, 180g steamed green beans	110g chicken breast, 180g green beans, salad with 1 tbsp olive oil and vinegar dressing	110g pork loin, saurkraut, 160g broccoli, 140g strawberries
snack 1	string cheese, apple	cheese, low-carbohydrate pretzels	110g cottage cheese with sliced peaches	string cheese, apple
snack 2	55g cottage cheese, diet fruit jelly	string cheese, 140g strawberries	string cheese, apple	200g plain yogurt

How does it work?

Achieved through changing one's diet to the optimal ratio of 40 per cent carbohydrate, 30 per cent fat, and 30 per cent protein, the so-called "zone" is a state where blood sugar levels are stable and hormonal balance is in equilibrium. Weight gain is triggered when the body finds itself outside of the "zone".

According to Sears, an excess of carbohydrates in diet produces an overabundance of insulin which can bring on cravings. This overload prompts the body to convert carbohydrates into fats and store them in your stomach, thighs, buttocks or other problem areas. Limiting the carbohydrates eaten and balancing them with 80–100g of low-fat protein at every meal keeps insulin and glucagon (a hormone produced by the pancreas that increases the level of sugar in the blood) on an even keel. This keeps hunger under control and the reduced number of calories produces weight loss. Meals should not exceed 500 calories and snacks should not exceed 100 calories.

Pros and cons

The Zone Diet promotes foods such as lean proteins, fresh vegetables, some fruits, leafy green vegetables and (primarily) monounsaturated fats. Some individuals, however, may find the recommended food combinations and working out the protein blocks challenging. Many foods are considered poor choices, so eating only the best might seem very limiting to some palates. Few foods have the naturally recommended proportions of carbohydrate,

weigh this up...
• No foods are completely off limits. You are allowed to eat anything as long as it has the right balance of proteins, carbs and fats. Foods are grouped as best, fair and poor choices.

fat and protein, so products such as ZonePerfect® bars and special ready-made dishes are available. Purchasing these products may increase the cost of following the Zone diet.

Is it for you?

Dieters who want a lower carbohydrate plan will like the Zone Diet; anyone who does not like preparing meals will appreciate ZonePerfect® bars. The programme would be tricky for busy families because of the time it takes to work out the appropriate food combinations.

Availability

Many common foods are either limited or considered poor choices. Special products, such as the ZonePerfect® bars, are recommended for optimum results.

Lifestyle changes

Regular exercise is recommended.

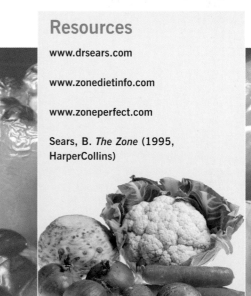

ratio of 40% carbohydrate, 30% fat and 30% protein.

wednesday	thursday	friday	**Resources**
porridge, 1 tbsp protein powder, soya milk, apple sauce, ½ slice bread, 2 tbsp peanut butter	pasturised egg substitute, cheese, 1 slice bread, 1⅓ tsp almond butter, 140g melon	porridge with 3 tbsp almonds, 240ml milk, egg, 50g blueberries	www.drsears.com
soya burger, 15g cheese, ½ hamburger bun, salad, 4 tsp olive oil and vinegar dressing	tuna salad with 4 tsp light mayonnaise in mini pitta pocket, 170g grapes	grilled chicken, Caesar salad, 1 tbsp Caesar dressing, ½ breadstick, 1 apple	www.zonedietinfo.com www.zoneperfect.com
stuffed red pepper, 100g chickpeas, onions, mushrooms, 30g cheese, 160g spinach, apple	110g chicken, onions, mushrooms, broccoli, mange-tout, 1½ tsp peanut oil, grapes	Lean Cuisine® fish fillet jardinière, 100g green beans, salad, 1 tbsp olive oil and vinegar dressing	**Sears, B.** *The Zone* (1995, HarperCollins)
cheese, 100g popcorn	string cheese, orange	440ml can of beer, 55g sliced turkey	
225ml milk	200g plain yogurt	225ml milk	

Note: All dairy produce is either low fat or fat free (yogurt, cheese, milk), breads are wholewheat, and the meat and poultry are lean.

CAMBRIDGE DIET

Originally a very low-calorie diet, the programme today emphasizes six steps to weight loss with different daily caloric recommendations.

Diet history

The diet originated from obesity research conducted in the 1960s and 1970s by Dr Alan Howard, a researcher at the University of Cambridge. Additional findings were then investigated by Dr Ian McLean-Baird. Today the Cambridge Diet is a global product with distributors all over the world.

How does it work?

This multi-step diet plan depends on specially devised, commercially branded accompanying products in the form of powder mixes combined with water or other liquids.

    The goal of the "Sole Source" programme (Step 1) is to achieve mild ketosis via the low intake of carbohydrates and calories so dieters are not allowed some of the sachets or Tetra Briks at this stage. As weight loss is achieved, calories (steps) are gradually increased until the individual reaches the weight maintenance phase (Step 6). Each client works with a certified Cambridge Counselor.

    The diet advocates four stages to success: preparation, weight loss, weight stabilization and weight maintenance. These coincide with the

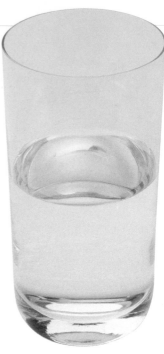

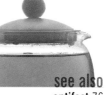

see also
optifast 76

LONG-TERM PLAN*

FLEXIBILITY*

FAMILY FRIENDLY

COST

STRENGTH OF SCIENCE

*EXCLUDES STEP 1

sample menu

This sample menu is in the style of the "Sole

	saturday	sunday	monday	tuesday
morning	Vanilla Sachet, black coffee, 360ml water	Banana Bliss Tetra Brik, black coffee, 360ml water	Butterscotch Sachet, black coffee, 360ml water	Banana Sachet, black coffee, 360ml water
lunch	Cappuccino Sachet, black tea, 360ml water	Chocolate Mint Sachet, black tea, 360ml water	Chocolate Velvet Tetra Brik, black tea, 360ml water	Fruits of the Forest Sachet, black tea, 360ml water
supper	Fruits of the Forest Sachet, black tea, 360ml water	Chicken and Mushroom Sachet, black tea, 360ml water	Vegetable Sachet, black tea, 360ml water	Chicken and Mushroom Sachet, black tea, 360ml water
snack 1	420ml water	420ml water	420ml water	420ml water
snack 2	420ml water	420ml water	420ml water	420ml water

six different steps: Step 1 – 415 to 554 calories a day for a maximum of 4 weeks at a time; Step 2 – 790 calories a day; Step 3 – 1,000 calories a day; Step 4 – 1,200 calories a day; Step 5 – 1,500 calories a day; and Step 6 – 1,500+ calories a day. The resulting weight loss is related to the low calorie intake so weight gain is likely to result once the person stops using the products and increases caloric intake once more.

Pros and cons

Each meal option is fortified to meet one-third of the recommended daily allowances for many vitamins and minerals but this can vary from country to country. An adequate consumption of fluids is strongly advised.

Steps 1 and 2 are quick-start, ultra-low-calorie, low-carbohydrate plans with little variety. Because most of the diet's counsellors start off as customers, they do not necessarily have a degree in nutrition. The plan's low calorie levels impede any long-term use as does the cost of the mixes and bars.

Is it for you?

It may appeal to someone who wants to lose weight but who may not have the time to measure out or prepare food and count calories. Anyone with a medical condition, on medication, pregnant or breast-feeding, children and adolescents should consult a doctor or a registered dietician. The Cambridge Diet will not be suitable for people who dislike depending on commercial products for weight loss.

weigh this up...
- Cambridge sachets contain a powder which, when mixed with hot or cold water, makes sweet-flavoured shakes or soups. Tetra Briks are ready-to-drink meal replacements. Both products are used as meal substitutes.

Availability

Although most of the foods in this diet are widely available from grocery shops and supermarkets, the Cambridge meals must come from a special distributor.

Lifestyle changes

Adjustments include substituting regular meals with specific branded Cambridge options and stopping eating out.

forbidden foods
- alcohol
- milky tea or coffee
- pure fruit juices
- sugary, high-calorie drinks

free foods
- black tea or coffee
- tap or bottled water (without fruit flavouring)

Source" programme, or Step 1.

wednesday	thursday	friday
Cappuccino Sachet, black coffee, 360ml water	Fruits of the Forest Sachet, black coffee, 360ml water	Strawberry Sachet, black coffee, 360ml water
Banana Bliss Tetra Brik, black tea, 360ml water	Chocolate Mint Sachet, black tea, 360ml water	Chicken and Mushroom Sachet, black tea, 360ml water
Vanilla Sachet, black tea, 360ml water	Vegetable Sachet, black tea, 360ml water	Banana Sachet, black tea, 360ml water
420ml water	420ml water	420ml water
420ml water	420ml water	420ml water

Resources

www.cambridge-diet.com

www.skinnyondiets.com

Howard, A. & Marks, J.
The Cambridge Diet: A Manual for Practitioners (1986, MTP Press)

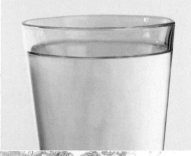

* The Cambridge "Sole Source" programme recommends 1,920ml of water. In addition to the water mixed in with the sachets, Tetra Briks, unsweetened black tea and unsweetened black coffee can be consumed daily.

LONG-TERM PLAN
● ● ●

FLEXIBILITY
● ●

FAMILY FRIENDLY
● ●

COST
●

STRENGTH OF SCIENCE
● ● ●

JENNY CRAIG DIET

Based on calorie and portion control, this weight-loss and maintenance programme fits your life by way of three key elements – your body, mind and relationship to food.

Diet history
Founded by Jenny Craig in 1983, the programme began in Australia and was introduced to the US in 1985. By 1987 Jenny Craig, Inc. had a total of 153 centres, including franchises in New Zealand and the United Kingdom. Currently there are 640 company-owned Jenny Craig Centres in the US, Canada, Australia, New Zealand, Guam and Puerto Rico. The corporation is now owned by Nestlé Nutrition.

How does it work?
The programme focuses on lifestyle factors for success: a healthy relationship to food, an active lifestyle and a balanced approach to living. Trained consultants are available at Jenny Craig centres for weekly one to one consultations (including a private weigh-in), on a helpline number or for live chat online. A variety of membership options and programmes are designed to meet the client's needs.

Although pre-packaged meals are an integral part of the weight loss incentive at the beginning, individuals are gradually encouraged to

weigh this up...
- You are allowed an unlimited amount of foods with 0–30 calories per serving, such as non-starchy vegetables and calorie-free drinks.
- Single-serve entrées help with portion control.

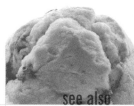

see also
nutrisystem 74
slim-fast 78
weight watchers 80

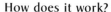

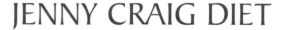

sample menu
This sample food plan follows the style of a Jenny

	saturday	sunday	monday	tuesday
morning	Banana Nut Muffin*, 1 medium fresh, peach, 240ml skimmed milk	Triple Grain Crisps*, 17 small grapes, 240ml skimmed milk	Breakfast Stuffed Sandwich*, 140g strawberries, 240ml skimmed milk	Complete Start Cereal*, 1 orange, 240ml skimmed milk
lunch	Italian Wedding Soup*, raw carrots, 100g garden salad, Jenny's Dressing*	Chicken Strips with, Rice Medley*, garden salad, Jenny's Dressing	Tuna Salad Kit*, garden salad, Jenny's Dressing*	Jenny's Personal Pizza*, garden salad, Jenny's Dressing*
supper	Turkey with Gravy*, 160g broccoli, MultiPlus*	Florentine Ravioli*, 140g summer squash, MultiPlus*	Meatloaf with BBQ Sauce*, 160g steamed courgettes, 1 tsp margarine, MultiPlus*	Salisbury Steak*, 160g cauliflower, MultiPlus*
snack 1	140g honeydew, Anytime Bar*	1 kiwi fruit, Anytime Bar* arugula salad with vinegar	110g fresh pineapple, Anytime Bar*	1 small apple, Anytime Bar*
snack 2	3 dates	1 small orange	½ large grapefruit	½ large pear
snack 3	Peanut Butter Bar*, 240ml skimmed milk	Lemon Cake*, 240ml skimmed milk	Bruschetta Veggie Chips*, 240ml skimmed milk	Trail Mix*, 240ml skimmed milk

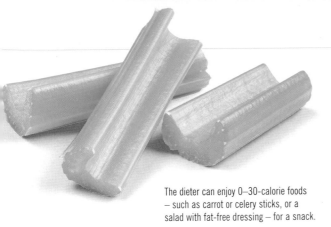

The dieter can enjoy 0–30-calorie foods – such as carrot or celery sticks, or a salad with fat-free dressing – for a snack.

decrease the frequency of these kinds of ready-made meals by learning to prepare lower calorie options in their quest to become educated about portion control. The strategy works by decreasing caloric intake and increasing physical activity. Strong scientific data supports this dual approach and its contribution to effective weight loss.

Pros and cons

Jenny Craig, Inc. offers an active 24/7 care and support operation for all its customers. The website offers inspirational recipes, tips and an interactive menu planner. There is also a medical advisory panel available to help – including a nutrition expert – but staff members are not registered dieticians. The pre-packaged meals can be expensive, especially if the cost is in addition to other family members' groceries. Once the pre-packaged meals are discontinued it can be challenging to maintain portion control.

Is it for you?

This diet plan will suit anyone with limited time and patience for counting calories and preparing meals. Anyone with a medical condition or who is pregnant should consult a physician before starting the programme. A child should not be put on it unless approved and monitored by a doctor or a registered dietician.

Availability

All of the food products in this diet can be bought at a local centre or ordered directly online.

Lifestyle changes

Increasing physical activity and becoming mindful of portion sizes are emphasized as daily activities.

healthy tips

- Choose fresh over tinned fruit to make the menu more nutrient dense.
- Limit certain kinds of foods – such as 100g cantaloupe, grapefruit, strawberries or watermelon (20–30 calories), and a piece of sugar-free chocolate (10–20 calories) – to no more than three servings a day.
- Drinking adequate water is also encouraged.
- Consumption of sugar-free gum is unlimited.

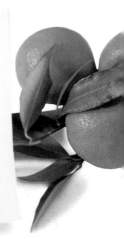

Craig 1,500 calorie menu.

wednesday	thursday	friday
Silver Dollar Pancakes and Veggie Sausage*, 70g blueberries, 240ml skimmed milk	Blueberry Muffin*, 1 small banana, 240ml skimmed milk	Sunshine Sandwich*, 140g raspberries, 240ml skimmed milk
Rotini with Meatballs*, garden salad, Jenny's Dressing*	Turkey Burger*, garden salad, Jenny's Dressing*, 1 small apple	Cheesy Enchiladas*, garden salad, Jenny's Dressing*
Sweet and Sour Chicken*, 150g carrots, 1 tsp margarine, MultiPlus*	Vegetable and Chicken Potstickers*, 180g green beans, MultiPlus*	Teriyaki Glazed Salmon*, 125g asparagus, MultiPlus*
1 small orange, Anytime Bar*, courgette, yellow squash	1 small plum, Anytime Bar*	⅓ small cantaloupe, Anytime Bar*
2 small tangerines	2 tbsp raisins	1 small nectarine
Sourdough Bites*, 240ml skimmed milk	Honey Oat Bar*, 240ml skimmed milk	Chocolate Chip Bites*, 240ml skimmed milk

Resources

www.jennycraig.com

Craig, J. *The Jenny Craig Story: How One Woman Changes Millions of Lives* (2004, John Wiley & Sons)

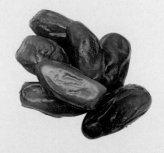

*Jenny Craig products. The menu includes three meals and three snacks daily with snacks consumed between mealtimes.

NUTRISYSTEM DIET

Based on the premise that lower glycaemic index foods promote weight loss, this program includes pre-packaged meals that are delivered directly to your doorstep.

LONG-TERM PLAN

FLEXIBILITY

FAMILY FRIENDLY
●●

COST
●

STRENGTH OF SCIENCE
●●●

Diet history

In 1972 the American company NutriSystem, Inc. began selling a liquid protein diet and made pre-packaged meals available to its customers only six years later. Although the company was officially declared bankrupt in the early 1990s and had to fold its weight-loss centre operation, nine years later it was globally accessible and selling its products to customers who ordered online.

How does it work?

Based around portion- and glycaemic-controlled meals for breakfast, lunch and dinner with at least one snack or dessert, the core meals of the NutriSystem programme are branded options plus any additional supplementary foods such as fresh fruit, vegetables and fat-free dairy products. Consuming plenty of water is also encouraged. Four individual programmes are offered, including menus specifically tailored for women, men, vegetarians and people with type 2 diabetes.

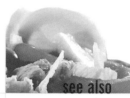

see also
gi 50
jenny craig 72
weight watchers 80

sample menu

This menu follows the style of the NutriSystem

	saturday	sunday	monday	tuesday
morning	Cranberry Orange Pastry*	Blueberry Muffin*	Apple Cinnamon Oatmeal*	Scrambled Egg Mix with Cheese*
lunch	Chicken Salad*	Tex-Mex Rice and Beans*	Balsamic Vinaigrette with Turkey Breast Meal*	Thousand Island Dressing with Chicken Breast*
supper	Vegetable Lasagne with Basil Tomato Sauce*	Rotini with Meatballs and Tomato Sauce*	Stroganoff Sauce with Beef and Noodles*	Chilli with Beans*
snack 1	Zesty Herb Snack Mix*	Strawberry Shortcake Bar*	Almond Biscotti*	BBQ Soy Chips*
snack 2	garden salad	small kiwi fruit	small banana	carrot sticks

The scientific evidence strongly supports the idea that making permanent and significant lifestyle changes, such as decreasing portions, controlling calories and increasing physical activity, promote effective weight loss. The general consensus, however, remains inconclusive about the effects of switching from pre-packaged meals to traditional eating and also about whether a low glycaemic index diet promotes weight loss.

Pros and cons

The four programmes available are varied with a different set of meal choices. NutriSystem's website has an interactive food log, exercise and journal component. Customers have access to 24/7 counselling services, both online and via telephone, to deal with weight-loss issues. The helpline counsellors are not registered dieticians, however, and the pre-packaged meals can be expensive to buy in the long run. Maintaining the appropriate portion control at mealtimes once the use of pre-packaged meals is discontinued can be challenging.

Is it for you?

The NutriSystem Diet is likely to suit individuals who have limited time available for calorie counting and meal preparation. Anyone with a medical condition or who is pregnant or breast-feeding should consult a doctor beforehand. A child should not be put on the programme unless his or her progress is being monitored by a doctor or a registered dietician.

healthy tips
• Supplement meals with a variety of fresh fruits, vegetables and fat-free dairy products.

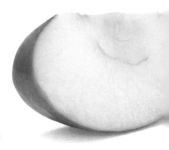

Availability

All the foods in this diet can only be bought online or by calling up a NutriSystem representative.

Lifestyle changes

Physical activity is actively encouraged.

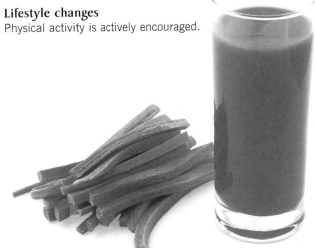

Nourish™ women's program.

	wednesday	thursday	friday
	Strawberry Toaster Pastry*	Peanut Butter Granola Bar*	Scrambled Eggs with Veggie Sausage Crumble*
	Black Beans and Ham Soup*	Cheese Tortellini*	Pasta with Beef*
	Beef Tacos*	Southwestern Style Chicken with Sauce*	Tuna Casserole*
	Chocolate Shake*	Pretzels*	Sour Cream and Onion Soy Chips*
	small apple	zucchini sticks	small orange

Resources

www.nutrisystem.com

www.glycemicindex.com

Rouse, J. *NutriSystem Nourish: The Revolutionary New Weight Loss Program* (2004, John Wiley & Sons)

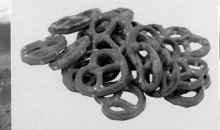

*NutriSystem products. Snack 1 would be referred to as "dessert" on this programme. NutriSystem, Inc. encourages the addition of fruits, vegetables and lower-fat or fat-free dairy options to meals and snacks. Drinking an adequate amount of water is strongly advised.

LONG-TERM PLAN

FLEXIBILITY

FAMILY FRIENDLY

COST

STRENGTH OF SCIENCE

OPTIFAST® PROGRAM

OPTIFAST is a weight-management programme that includes medical, behavioural and nutritional interventions. The formula diet is portion controlled and calorie restricted.

Diet history
Owned by Novartis Nutrition, the OPTIFAST full meal replacement programme began in 1974. It was the first comprehensive formula diet programme designed for the treatment of obesity. Today, OPTIFAST clinics are located in the US, Canada, Australia and Spain.

How does it work?
The Active Weight Loss Phase, or full-formula phase, consists of consuming only OPTIFAST meal replacement products. Since these products are portion and calorie controlled, this phase is a low-calorie diet. The next phase, which lasts about six weeks, is a transition period. During this time, self-prepared foods and meals are brought back into the diet. This is followed by the Long-Term Management Diet, which includes foods like fruit, vegetables, grains and low-fat proteins, along with OPTIFAST meal replacement products.

The programme combines education, to help with lifestyle changes, with a fully nutritionally complete, formula-controlled diet that is monitored by a doctor. The calorie amounts throughout the programme usually vary from 800–1,500 calories per day. There is strong scientific data to support the theory that a decrease in calories promotes weight loss, and that behaviour modification will help sustain it.

see also
cambridge 70

sample menu
A typical menu plan during the Active Weight

	saturday	sunday	monday	tuesday
breakfast	OPTIFAST 800 Vanilla Powder drink	OPTIFAST 800 Strawberry Ready to Drink	OPTIFAST 800 French Vanilla Ready to Drink	OPTIFAST 800 Chocolate Powder drink
mid-morning	OPTIFAST 800 Strawberry Powder drink	OPTIFAST 800 Chocolate Powder drink	OPTIFAST 800 Garden Tomato Powder Soup	OPTIFAST 800 Strawberry Ready to Drink
lunch	OPTIFAST 800 French Vanilla Ready to Drink	OPTIFAST 800 Garden Tomato Powder Soup	OPTIFAST 800 Chocolate Ready to Drink	OPTIFAST 800 Chicken Powder Soup
mid-afternoon	OPTIFAST 800 Chocolate Powder drink	OPTIFAST 800 Strawberry Powder drink	OPTIFAST 800 Vanilla Powder drink	OPTIFAST 800 Chocolate Ready to Drink
supper	OPTIFAST 800 Chicken Powder Soup	OPTIFAST 800 French Vanilla Ready to Drink	OPTIFAST 800 Strawberry Powder drink	OPTIFAST 800 Vanilla Powder drink
snack 1	OPTIFAST Nutrition Bar	OPTIFAST Nutrition Bar	OPTIFAST Nutrition Bar	OPTIFAST Nutrition Bar

Pros and cons

This is a customized multi-disciplinary team approach to weight loss and management. Medical monitoring is provided to participants, and the website has an excellent Wellness Toolbox section with resource links. Upon completion of the programme, the participant is encouraged to participate in an ongoing long-term management programme.

However, the selection of products may become monotonous for some. The meal replacement products can be expensive. Once they are discontinued, maintaining the appropriate portion control with homemade meals may prove challenging and the weight lost may be regained.

Is it for you?

It is likely to appeal those who have limited time for counting calories and meal preparation. Medical screening and examination is done by the programme doctor prior to starting the Active Weight Loss Phase. This phase is not appropriate for a child or for a woman who is pregnant or breast-feeding. Some bariatric surgeons will recommend the diet to patients who are not candidates for surgery.

weigh this up...
- During the Active Weight Loss Phase, spend time learning about portion control and calorie amounts to make the transition easier.

Availability

OPTIFAST products can be purchased only through an OPTIFAST provider, due to the medical supervision required and the low-calorie option. Total food cost will vary if the dieter must buy other foods for the family.

Lifestyle changes

The programme encourages exercise. It also includes nutrition education and other behaviour modification techniques and resources.

note
The information given here is based on the US OPTIFAST Program. There may be differences between this programme and those run in other countries – please check the website below for further details.

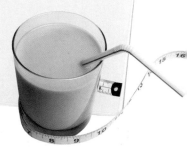

Loss Phase – flavours and type of drink can be varied to taste.

wednesday	thursday	friday
OPTIFAST 800 Strawberry Powder drink	OPTIFAST 800 Vanilla Powder drink	OPTIFAST 800 Strawberry Ready to Drink
OPTIFAST 800 Chocolate Ready to Drink	OPTIFAST 800 French Vanilla Ready to Drink	OPTIFAST 800 Chocolate Powder drink
OPTIFAST 800 Vanilla Powder drink	OPTIFAST 800 Chocolate Ready to Drink	OPTIFAST 800 Garden Tomato Powder Soup
OPTIFAST 800 Chicken Powder Soup	OPTIFAST 800 Strawberry Powder drink	OPTIFAST 800 French Vanilla Ready to Drink
OPTIFAST 800 Garden Tomato Powder Soup	OPTIFAST 800 Chicken Powder Soup	OPTIFAST 800 Vanilla Powder drink
OPTIFAST Nutrition Bar	OPTIFAST Nutrition Bar	OPTIFAST Nutrition Bar

Resources

www.optifast.com

www.optifast.com/bookshelf.do

For the Spanish clinic:
http://nc.novartisconsumerhealth.es

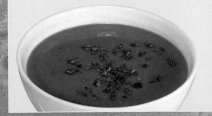

Note: In Active Weight Loss Phase, two **OPTIFAST** Bar servings can replace one **OPTIFAST** 800 serving. No more than two servings of **OPTIFAST** 800 Soup should be consumed per day due to sodium content.

LONG-TERM PLAN

FLEXIBILITY

FAMILY FRIENDLY

COST

STRENGTH OF SCIENCE

SLIM-FAST

This mostly liquid, partial meal replacement plan includes shakes for breakfast and lunch, plus bars for snacking in between meals.

Diet history
The original concept was born of research using a liquid formula meal. Metrical™, the first meal replacement formula, was commercially available for weight reduction back in the 1950s. Similar products have come and gone over the years but Slim-Fast is a popular meal replacement today.

How does it work?
If followed attentively, this diet promises an average weight drop of about 1kg (2lb) per week. The programme recommends one Slim-Fast shake in a can for breakfast followed by another one for lunch plus 200 calories from a chosen food, fruit or vegetable and a sensible healthy dinner in the evening of up to 600 calories. To help maintain your energy levels you can snack up to two times a day and make sure you drink around two litres of water to avoid dehydration.

The amount of extra calories allowed at lunchtime will depend on the gap between the individual's actual weight and his or her weight-loss goal. Two Slim-Fast snack bars are recommended between meals for "on-the-go" busy people. "Forbidden" meals include the usual breakfast and lunch. Alternative dinner recipes are suggested and

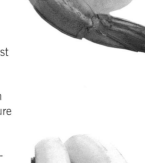

see also
jenny craig 72
weight watchers 80

sample menu
For people on the go, shakes and bars provide a

	saturday	sunday	monday	tuesday
morning	Slim-Fast Optima Shake	Slim-Fast Optima Shake	Slim-Fast Optima Shake	Slim-Fast Optima Shake
lunch	Slim-Fast Optima Shake, 200g fruit yogurt, water	Slim-Fast Optima Shake, 110g cottage cheese with fruit, diet cola	Slim-Fast Optima Shake, 1 slice cheese, 1 slice bread, diet cola	Slim-Fast Optima Shake, 110g cottage cheese with fruit, water
supper	rice, grilled tofu, three-bean salad, vegetable medley, spring green salad, orange and banana	Spanish rice with soya meat and seafood, spinach and strawberry salad, carrot cake, berries, water	roast beef, baked potato, green beans, carrots, tossed salad, fruit, yogurt, water	prawns with onion, garlic and basil, with pasta, cucumber and tomato salad, bread, diet cola
snack 1	Slim-Fast Optima Bar, ⅛ melon	Slim-Fast Optima Muffin Bar, 50g blueberries	Slim-Fast Optima Bar, apple	Slim-Fast Optima Bar, banana
snack 2	Slim-Fast Optima Muffin Bar, ½ grapefruit	Slim-Fast Optima Bar, ⅛ melon	Slim-Fast Optima Bar, banana	Slim-Fast Optima Bar, orange

healthy, low-calorie frozen meals are recommended. Vegetables and fruit are encouraged either with dinner or snacks.

If the plan is followed with controlled dinner portions, the day's meals and snacks come to about 1,500 calories. The plan strongly discourages the consumption of empty calories such as sweets and crisps. Along with the recommended amount of exercise, it causes a calorie deficit while providing the essential nutrients.

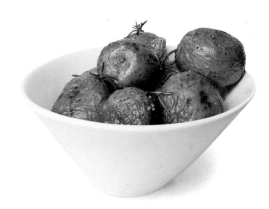

Pros and cons

There is some scientific evidence to indicate that the Slim-Fast Diet is more effective than other calorie-controlled competitors. The plan encourages exercise, high-fibre foods, allows for an unlimited amount of calorie-free drinks, and provides a list of specific lean meat products, vegetables and starch choices.

A noticeable drawback is a high drop-out rate, probably due to lack of meals and the monotony of liquid meal replacements. Canned shakes, bars, and snacks are conveniently packaged but more expensive than regular food. There may not be sufficient variety in food intake which will tend to be low in fibre unless enough fruit and vegetables are eaten.

Is it for you?

This diet may appeal to individuals who have busy lifestyles which allow no time for home cooking or the fresh preparation of meals. There is a general disclaimer to check with your doctor before going on the Slim-Fast Plan Diet but the plan is generally suitable for all people, except young children, pregnant women or women who are breast-feeding.

Availability

Slim-Fast products are widely available nationwide from most general food stores and supermarkets.

Lifestyle changes

Exercise is strongly recommended as part of the programme. Tips are available on using smaller serving plates or bowls, on eating slowly so you feel fuller on less, and on avoiding fat-free products that are full of sugar.

quick no-prep meal replacement.

wednesday	thursday	friday	**Resources**
Slim-Fast Optima Shake	Slim-Fast Optima Shake	Slim-Fast Optima Shake	www.Slim.Fast.com
Slim-Fast Optima Shake, 220g fruit yogurt, water	Slim-Fast Optima Shake, 30g turkey, 1 slice bread, diet soda	Slim-Fast Optima Shake, 1 slice cheese, 1 slice bread, diet cola	Hutton, L., Kotz, D. *The Slim-Fast Body, Mind, Life Makeover* (2000, HarperCollins)
grilled chicken, roasted new potatoes, peas, corn, carrots, green salad, mixed fruit, water	roast turkey slices, rice, grilled asparagus, cauliflower and red pepper salad, water	grilled salmon steaks, wild rice, mushroom sauce, broccoli, carrots, stewed prunes and apricots, diet cola	
Slim-Fast Optima Muffin Bar, 10 grapes	Slim-Fast Optima Bar, orange	Slim-Fast Optima Muffin Bar, 6 strawberries	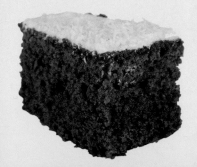
Slim-Fast Optima Muffin Bar, 10 grape tomatoes	Slim-Fast Optima Muffin Bar, 6 strawberries	Slim-Fast Optima Bar, orange	

Note: Slim-Fast Optima shakes, bars and muffins are branded products. All yogurts, soft or cottage cheeses and dressings should be fat free. All grains, breads and pasta should be whole grain or wholewheat.

WEIGHT WATCHERS

The Weight Watchers approach is built on four pillars – making wise food choices, regular physical activity, developing cognitive skills and a supportive environment.

LONG-TERM PLAN

FLEXIBILITY

FAMILY FRIENDLY

COST

STRENGTH OF SCIENCE

Diet history

Weight Watchers was started by Jean Nidetch, a woman tired of unsuccessful diet regimes. She started meeting regularly with other overweight friends to create a support system. Word spread, and the number of participants grew. Weight Watchers, Inc. began officially in May 1963, with 400 attendees. Jean Nidetch and her partners sold the company to HJ Heinz Co. in 1978. Weight Watchers International, Inc. has over 1.5 million members attending one of its 50,000 weekly meetings around the world. In the 1970s Weight Watchers incorporated a walking programme and became one of the first weight-loss programmes to emphasize physical activity. Today one can purchase Weight Watchers food products as well as a variety of other products, including magazines and exercise tapes.

How does it work?

The original Weight Watchers food plan evolved over the years, going from a "diet sheet" to an exchange system. In 1998, the exchange system was replaced with the POINTS® Weight-Loss System, which assigns a POINTS value to activities and to food, determined by the number of calories, total fat and dietary fibre in a defined serving. Based on a personalized quiz, each person is

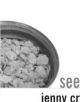

see also
jenny craig 72
nutrisystem 74
slim-fast 78

sample menu

A sample seven-day food plan in the style of the

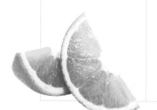

	saturday	sunday	monday	tuesday
morning	50g vanilla puffed wheat, 1 glass skimmed milk, 100g strawberries, 1 slice wholewheat bread, 1 tsp margarine	egg, ham, and cheese sandwich on scone, skinny latte	70g cinnamon toast crunch cereal, 1 glass skimmed milk, 240ml orange juice	egg bagel, ½ medium cantaloupe, ½ glass skimmed-milk latte
lunch	grilled chicken breast, red pepper strips, brown rice, grapes	grilled cheese sandwich, tossed side salad, 1 tbsp Italian salad dressing	80g light tuna, baby greens, cherry tomatoes, low-calorie dressing, vegetable crackers	small hamburger, green salad with no-calorie dressing, apple, ½ glass skimmed milk
supper	noodle bowl, Thai-style chicken, egg-drop soup, chicory salad	tuna noodle casserole, shredded savoy cabbage	oven-fried chicken parmesan, grilled aubergine, hard roll, salad, no-calorie dressing, pear	chicken lo mein, steamed snow peas, 100g blueberries
snack 1*	English toffee crunch bar	140g strawberries, lemon angel cake	strawberry-banana smoothie	skinny vanilla non-fat yogurt
snack 2*	non-fat strawberry yogurt	blueberries and cream yogurt	Weight Watchers chocolate mousse bar	chocolate round ice cream sandwich

given a daily POINTS Target that will lead to a caloric deficit that translates into a ½–1kg (1–2lb) per week weight loss (after the first three weeks when weight loss may be greater due to water loss). In 2004, another food plan was added, the Core Plan®, which focuses on choosing foods with a low energy density. By routinely monitoring hunger cues and with an allowance for periodic "indulgences", the Core Plan has been shown to lead to weight losses equal to the POINTS System. Both plans share the Good Health Guidelines – eight recommendations that ensure the food choices made are nutritionally sound and meet current nutrition recommendations. Members are rewarded with a 10 per cent weight loss and Lifetime Membership is awarded when a healthy body weight (i.e., BMI 20–25 or as prescribed by a qualified healthcare provider) is achieved and a six-week maintenance plan is completed. Support and accountability are keys to success and are provided at weekly meetings and weigh-ins.

Pros and cons

There is strong evidence to support that a lifestyle plan that includes regular monitoring and support systems using commonly available foods can be successful in weight management. The emphasis on portion control and low energy density foods can be translated to many food-related settings and the recipes can teach dieters to prepare many dishes lower in calories than their usual counterparts. Dieters can also subscribe to an online version – Weight Watchers Online. Members do have to pay for weight-loss services, including those on the Internet.

Is it for you?

This diet will appeal to those who need a strong support network and want to learn how to manage weight using a successful lifelong plan. Individuals can also sign up and participate in a programme through the official website. The plan's focus is on variety and portion control across food categories and is not likely to harm anyone. It may not be ideal for someone who cannot or does not want to participate in physical activities, follow a structured food plan or talk about weight-related issues.

It will appeal to persons who need a support system and want to learn how to manage weight using a lifelong plan. The plan includes variety and portion control, but may be difficult for persons who cannot participate in some of the support activities, which are an important part of the plan. The plan is not likely to harm dieters, but a person who is not interested in or does not like to participate in physical activity, follow a rigid food plan or talk to others about weight issues may have difficulty adhering to the plan.

Availability

Dieters can follow Weight Watchers using general foods purchased. Weight Watchers branded foods are also available as a convenience.

Lifestyle changes

Weight Watchers was one of the first programmes to incorporate physical activity and a cognitive behaviour system into its plan.

Weight Watchers POINTS® Food System (1,050–1,400 calories).

wednesday	thursday	friday	Resources
			www.weightwatchers.com
50g bran flakes, 1 glass skimmed milk, 1 apple	230ml pineapple juice, scrambled egg substitute, baked hash browns, skinny latte	25g Honey Bunches of Oats cereal, 1 glass skimmed milk, ½ grapefruit	
low-fat cottage cheese and orange sections, 10 mild cheddar biscuits	grilled salmon, 110g rice, 60g vegetable stir-fry	peanut butter and raisin sandwich, 1 glass skimmed milk, pear	
fiesta fajita chicken, steamed green beans, green salad, no-calorie Italian dressing	mandarin chicken, steamed carrots, sugarsnap peas	pork loin chop, courgettes, mashed potatoes	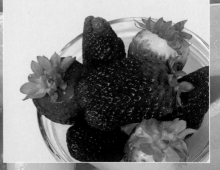
skinny vanilla sundae cup	orange, mild cheddar stick	low-calorie brownie bar with fudge filling	
fat-free carrot cake	skinny decaffinated latte	1 glass pineapple juice	

*Some of these snacks are commercial Weight Watchers products.

LONG-TERM PLAN

FLEXIBILITY

FAMILY FRIENDLY

COST
●

STRENGTH OF SCIENCE
●●

3-APPLE-A-DAY PLAN

This strategy includes an apple as part of each meal. Participants are encouraged to follow the meal plan, increase water intake and start walking.

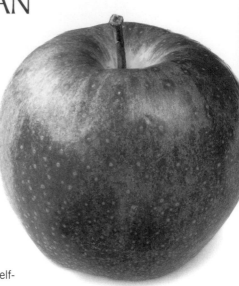

Diet history
Registered dietician, Tammi Flynn, developed this plan from watching her weight-loss clients at a health club over several years. She noticed a connection between those who ate a lot of apples and a higher amount of fat loss. From the success she observed in her clients, the 3-Apple-a-Day Plan was penned into a whole eating strategy, complete with meal plans. The book was originally self-published in 2003 and re-published in 2005.

How does it work?
Eating a fresh apple before each meal can help curb appetite, prevent overeating and promote weight loss. Apples are a good source of fibre. Eating an apple before each meal helps the dieter to feel fuller and, hopefully, consume fewer calories. There are many health benefits associated with eating apples and, more specifically, a high-fibre diet,

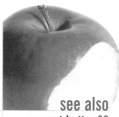

see also
peanut butter 92
volumetrics 108

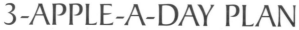

sample menu

Each meal in this plan should include an apple in

	saturday	sunday	monday	tuesday
morning	apple, breakfast burrito	apple, devilled eggs, fat-free muffin	apple, omelette with meat and cheese	apple, Southwest scrambled eggs, instant porridge
lunch	apple, homemade chilli	apple, rice with cooked turkey, cooked broccoli	apple, 2 chicken breasts, steamed broccoli, brown rice	apple, turkey burger with cheese on wholegrain bun, cooked vegetables
supper	Waldorf salad	Southwest salad, baked apple dessert	apple, green salad with salmon	apple, grilled chicken with tossed salad
snack 1	homemade fruit smoothie	wholegrain crackers with salmon	fat-free cottage cheese and fat-free yogurt	protein shake
snack 2	homemade fruit shake	homemade vanilla shake	coffee-flavoured nutrition shake	fat-free, lightly-flavoured yogurt

including lowering cholesterol, bowel movement regularity, cancer prevention and lower risk of heart disease.

The author discusses how to improve overall diet and strongly encourages increased exercise and water consumption. There are no calorie restrictions or counting.

Pros and cons

This plan is simple in that the main change is adding three apples to the daily diet. Apples are always available in many varieties. Because apples are portable, this is also great for those who are out and about or on the go most of the day.

However, increasing fibre intake too quickly may cause some intestinal discomfort. Some people may grow tired of eating three apples a day.

Is it for you?

This plan is suitable for those looking for a simple and healthy weight-loss plan. It is not appropriate for anyone who is allergic to apples or those who have to consume a low-fibre diet due to a medical condition.

Availability

Apples are available year-round at any grocery shop. The other foods in the diet are those the person would usually buy and eat.

Lifestyle changes

Exercise is a crucial component of this plan. The author stresses the importance of exercising regularly and incorporating weight training to promote fat loss. Other changes emphasized are a low-fat diet and drinking 8–10 glasses of water a day.

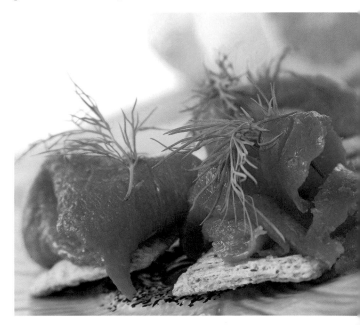

some form.

wednesday	thursday	friday
porridge with apple slices	apple, high-fibre cereal with fat-free milk	apple, omelette with vegetables and cheese
apple, lasagne with minced turkey, green salad with fat-free dressing	apple, meat stew	apple, wholewheat spaghetti with marinara sauce
stir-fry with chicken, vegetables and apple chunks	apple, tuna with green salad	apple, Caesar salad topped with grilled salmon
homemade fruit smoothie	celery with peanut butter	low-fat cottage cheese, skimmed milk
coffee-flavoured nutrition shake	homemade fruit smoothie	homemade chocolate shake

Resources

www.3appleplan.com

www.getfitfoods.com/3-apple.cfm

Flynn, T. *The 3-Apple-a-Day Plan* (2005, Broadway Books)

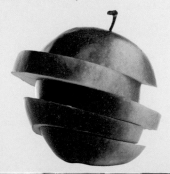

LONG-TERM PLAN

FLEXIBILITY

FAMILY FRIENDLY

COST

STRENGTH OF SCIENCE

NEW CABBAGE SOUP DIET

This one-week plan includes cabbage soup and, depending on the day, a variety of other foods.

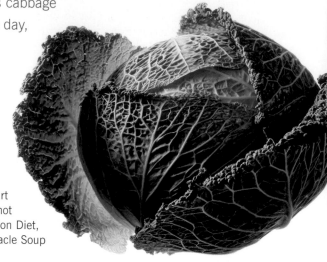

Diet history

The New Cabbage Soup diet was published in 1997 but variations of a Cabbage Soup Diet have been around for several years. This includes plans such as the Fat-Burning Soup Diet, Sacred Heart Hospital Diet (not affiliated with any of the existing Sacred Heart Hospitals), New Mayo Clinic Diet (not part of The Mayo Clinic), Dolly Parton Diet, Military Cabbage Soup, and TJ Miracle Soup Diet (which it is not).

How does it work?

This is recommended as a seven-day, quick weight-loss plan. Some variations recommend it for one week, alternating for two weeks with a maintenance plan and a repeat of the one-week quick plan.

The plan provides some weight loss due to its low-calorie content and limited food choices. In addition to soup, the menus include a

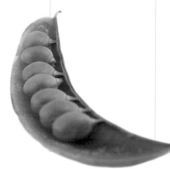

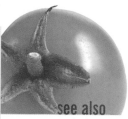

see also
grapefruit 88

sample menu
This plan allows unlimited amounts of cabbage

	saturday	sunday	monday	tuesday
morning	240g yogurt, coffee	smoothie with 240g yogurt, blueberries and strawberries, coffee	120g yogurt , 200g mixed berries, coffee	120g yogurt, sliced cucumber with parsley, tea
lunch	cabbage soup, grilled chicken breast, grilled asparagus, aubergine and courgette	cabbage soup, greens, carrot slices, peas, radishes, broccoli and cauliflower salad, low-calorie dressing	cabbage soup, baked apple, tea	cabbage soup, mixed vegetables, coffee
supper	cabbage soup, grilled fish, sugar-snap peas, sliced beetroot, mixed greens with low-fat dressing	cabbage soup, steamed green beans, boiled parsnips, baked apple rings	cabbage soup, orange and grapefruit wedges, tea	cabbage soup, large baked potato with 120g yogurt, herbed squash and green beans, water
snack 1	water, cucumber and carrot sticks	tea, honeydew and cantaloupe salad	tea, 120g yogurt, canteloupe	water, 100g yogurt, carrot sticks
snack 2	cabbage soup, cherry tomatoes	water, 240g yogurt, pear and apple slices	water, banana	cabbage soup

serving of dairy, fruit and/or vegetables, and low- or no-fat dressing. However, if skimmed milk is consumed with coffee in the morning, yogurt is not allowed until later in the day. Days five and six include chicken or fish.

In a prototype of the older version of the diet, days one to four consist of unlimited amounts of cabbage soup, fruit and/or vegetables. Day five includes cabbage soup, some meat or chicken and tomatoes. Day seven includes cabbage soup, brown rice and vegetables. Unsweetened coffee, tea, cranberry juice or water are allowed daily.

The plan allows unlimited soup, so not restricting the amount eaten may appeal to some, but, in reality, the monotony is likely to limit their food and caloric intake. This is basically a low-calorie, low-fat diet with some fibre from the cabbage and other vegetables and fruit. The fluid content from soup is likely to promote a feeling of fullness, but claims that the cabbage soup itself has fat-burning properties are not supported by scientific evidence. There are variations of, and recipes for, the diet available through the Internet.

Pros and cons

The diet is simple and easy to remember and follow, with one main food. It is low in calories for the short term, so it will produce temporary weight loss.

Although some other vegetables are included, as well as fruit, the plan's focus on one food will inevitably make it monotonous. The high amounts of cabbage may cause uncomfortable flatulence levels, and some may feel distended or bloated. The restrictions on many foods makes the plan low on several nutrients, such as protein and carbohydrates, and it should not be followed for more than one week. Eating out will be difficult, or impossible, unless the restaurant has cabbage soup or dieters can take their own soup.

Is it for you?

This will appeal to those who like large amounts of cabbage (and soup) and do not mind eating them daily for about one week.

Pregnant women, the frail, elderly, persons with special conditions (such as diabetes), or individuals with gastrointestinal disorders (such as irritable bowel syndrome) or colitis first need to consult a doctor and work closely with a registered dietician to determine if they should try this diet, and how best to use it.

Availability

The foods are available in a general food shop.

Lifestyle changes

Generally none, but some plans recommend drinking lots of water.

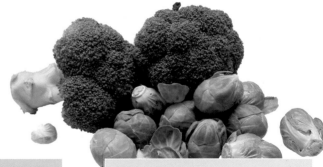

soup with some daily variations.

	wednesday	thursday	friday
	skimmed milk, strawberry and banana smoothie	240g yogurt, 2 bananas, coffee	120g yogurt, coffee
	cabbage soup, steamed carrots, cos lettuce with calorie-free Caesar dressing, tea	cabbage soup, 2 glasses skimmed milk, 2 bananas	cabbage soup, grilled fish with 260g crushed tomatoes, water
	cabbage soup, spinach salad, orange slices and citrus low-calorie dressing	cabbage soup, 2 glasses skimmed milk	cabbage soup, grilled chicken breast with 3 grilled tomatoes, water
	tea, mixed fruit salad	skimmed milk, baked banana	water, grilled, herbed chicken strips
	water, celery sticks	skimmed milk and banana smoothie	tea, 120g yogurt

Note: Use plain, non-fat yogurt.

Resources

www.cabbage-soup-diet.com

www.napa.ufl.edu/2002news/cabbagediet.htm

Danbrot, M. *The New Cabbage Soup Diet* (2004, St. Martin's Press)

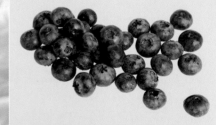

LONG-TERM PLAN

FLEXIBILITY

FAMILY FRIENDLY

COST

STRENGTH OF SCIENCE

DRINKING MAN'S DIET

One of the original ultra-low carbohydrate, weight-loss programmes to hit the mainstream.

Diet history

The Drinking Man's Diet, first published by Robert Cameron in 1964, has sold over 2.4 million copies worldwide and been translated into 13 languages.

How does it work?

The rationale behind the Drinking Man's Diet is that the total amount of carbohydrates consumed should be limited to 60g per day, as they are immediately turned by the body into fat when present in excess. The diet allows proteins and fats to be consumed during the day as they provide satiety – a vital factor for any diet's success rate.

Since most alcoholic beverages contain minimal carbohydrate content, they are incorporated into a plan which purports noticeable results within days. It claims that weight loss is possible because carbohydrates are converted into fat while the calories in proteins and fats are invariably metabolized. Such a drastic reduction in carbohydrates, however, means a big dip in the number of daily calories allowed. The body of scientific evidence contradicts the diet's central tenet because once the body's caloric requirements are exceeded, any kind of food is converted to fat.

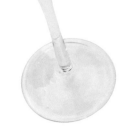

Most of the calories in a martini come from the alcohol, not carbohydrates.

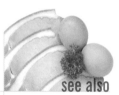

see also
atkins 42

sample menu

The Drinking Man's Diet encourages low-carb

	saturday	sunday	monday	tuesday
morning	cantaloupe, eggs and bacon, coffee	blueberries, sausage and eggs, coffee	cantaloupe, ham and eggs, coffee	tomato juice, bacon and eggs, coffee
lunch	salad with Roquefort dressing, chicken	pork fillet with broccoli and carrots	lettuce and tomato salad with olive oil dressing, steak, asparagus	salad with Roquefort dressing, pork loin, tea
supper	sea bass with carrots and peas, gin and tonic (if desired)	lettuce and tomato salad with olive oil dressing, leg of lamb, rum and diet cola (if desired)	artichoke with aubergine and ham, martini (if desired)	lettuce and tomato salad with olive oil dressing, halibut, wine (if desired)
snack 1	cured ham, cheese, burgundy	olives, salami, martini	cheese, red wine	cashews, martini
snack 2	prawn cocktail	sardines	prawn cocktail	popcorn

weigh this up...

- How much alcohol can you really have? One unit of alcohol or one drink is defined as 350ml of a regular beer (about 150 calories), 150ml of wine (about 100 calories) or 40ml of 40% spirit (about 100 calories).
- Low-carbohydrate alcoholic drinks are permitted in this diet. You can drink in moderation during mealtimes because alcohol consumption during digestion allows for a slower rate of absorption.

healthy tips

- Avoid cutting out carbs completely!
- Familiarize yourself with the grams per servings in different sources of vegetables, fruits and grains.
- Include nutrient-rich vegetables, such as dark green and dark orange vegetables, in your daily diet.
- How many grams of carbohydrates can you have? Approximately 100g rice, hot cereal, or starchy vegetables, 1 slice bread or 1 serving of fruit.

Pros and cons

The diet claims minimal effort is required to lose a substantial amount of weight. It allows you to eat foods with trace amounts of carbohydrates (such as beef, chicken, veal, turkey, lamb, *foie gras*, martinis, spirits, and any fruits and vegetable) in liberal quantities. Since many kinds of carbohydrates are restricted, however, the dieter may end up deficient in fibre and certain vitamins and minerals. Conclusive scientific evidence about the effects of such a diet on cardiovascular health is still not available.

Is it for you?

This diet will appeal to healthy individuals who do power or business lunches, or enjoy socializing and sitting down to rich meals and drinks low in carbohydrates. Anyone with a medical condition must first consult a doctor.

Availability

Although this diet caters to the expensive tastes of fine-dining business executives, it can be also be followed using everyday foods from your local supermarket.

Lifestyle changes

None suggested.

foods and moderate consumption of alcohol.

	wednesday	thursday	friday
	grapefruit, sausage and eggs, tea	honeydew, eggs and steak	tomato slices, ham and cheese slices
	green beans, kale, lobster tail	salad with Roquefort dressing, roast duck	salmon, Brussels sprouts, cauliflower
	lettuce and tomato salad with olive oil dressing, steak, cocktail (if desired)	creamed spinach, lamb chops, cordial (if desired)	lettuce and tomato salad with olive oil dressing, chicken, Manhattan (if desired)
	turkey, cheese, pinot grigio	cucumber with balsamic vinegar	cheese, red wine
	pistachios	steamed mussels	martini, olives, cheese

Resources

Jameson, G. and Williams, E. *The Drinking Man's Diet* (2004, revised ed. Cameron & Co.)

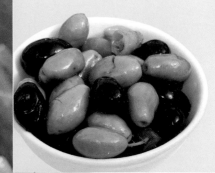

LONG-TERM PLAN

FLEXIBILITY

FAMILY FRIENDLY

COST
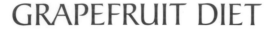

STRENGTH OF SCIENCE

GRAPEFRUIT DIET

This calorie-restricted plan favours vitamin-rich grapefruit to promote a healthy body weight.

Diet history

One of the oldest known fad diets, it emerged as the "Hollywood Diet" during the glamorous 1930s and regained popularity when grapefruit consumption once again became associated with weight reduction as part of the Grapefruit Diet Plan. You can find variations of the plan on the Internet. In the past it has been wrongly referred to as the Mayo Clinic Diet.

How does it work?

This low-calorie plan is easy to follow and is recommended for kickstarting quick weight loss as you eat three meals and enjoy a daily snack in addition to having grapefruit with every meal.

Although grapefruit is credited with a special fat-burning enzyme, these claims remain scientifically unfounded. The body of research so far credits the weight loss with a limited food selection, reduced caloric intake and loss of fluid. Complex carbohydrates and snacks between meals are forbidden but most vegetables and all meat and fish are allowed. Meals are comprised of eggs, meat or fish, salads, vegetables, skimmed milk, tomato juice and unlimited amounts of black coffee or tea. Accompany each meal with half a grapefruit or half a cup of unsweetened grapefruit juice.

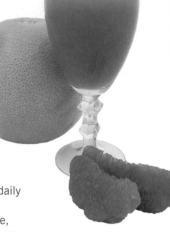

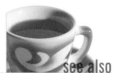

see also
new cabbage soup 84

sample menu

Each meal includes half a grapefruit or half a cup

	saturday	sunday	monday	tuesday
morning	½ grapefruit or 120ml grapefruit juice (unsweetened), 2 eggs (any style), 2 slices bacon, black coffee or tea	½ grapefruit or 120ml grapefruit juice (unsweetened), 2 eggs (any style), 2 slices bacon, black coffee or tea	½ grapefruit or 120ml grapefruit juice (unsweetened), 2 eggs (any style), 2 slices bacon, black coffee or tea	½ grapefruit or 120ml grapefruit juice (unsweetened), 2 eggs (any style), 2 slices bacon, black coffee or tea
lunch	½ grapefruit or 120ml grapefruit juice (unsweetened), meat or fish (any style or amount), salad with low-fat or no-fat dressing, black coffee or tea	½ grapefruit or 120ml grapefruit juice (unsweetened), meat or fish (any style or amount), salad with low-fat or no-fat dressing, black coffee or tea	½ grapefruit or 120ml grapefruit juice (unsweetened), meat or fish (any style or amount), salad with low-fat or no-fat dressing, black coffee or tea	½ grapefruit or 120ml grapefruit juice (unsweetened), meat or fish (any style or amount), salad with low-fat or no-fat dressing, black coffee or tea
supper	½ grapefruit or 120ml grapefruit juice (unsweetened), meat or fish (any style, any amount), vegetables (any green, yellow or red vegetables cooked in butter or with any seasoning), black coffee or tea	½ grapefruit or 120ml grapefruit juice (unsweetened), meat or fish (any style, any amount), vegetables (any green, yellow or red vegetables cooked in butter or with any seasoning), black coffee or tea	½ grapefruit or 120ml grapefruit juice (unsweetened), meat or fish (any style, any amount), vegetables (any green, yellow or red vegetables cooked in butter or with any seasoning), black coffee or tea	½ grapefruit or 120ml grapefruit juice (unsweetened), meat or fish (any style, any amount), vegetables (any green, yellow or red vegetables cooked in butter or with any seasoning), black coffee or tea
snack	1 glass tomato juice or 1 glass skimmed milk	1 glass tomato juice or 1 glass skimmed milk	1 glass tomato juice or 1 glass skimmed milk	1 glass tomato juice or 1 glass skimmed milk

This 12-day diet plan and 1,000-calorie daily menu are reputed to help you lose a minimum of 4½kg (10lb) Meals are low in carbohydrates but include meat, fish, high-protein or high-fat foods, salad, vegetables and unlimited amounts of black coffee or tea. Modified versions of the plan also introduce fruit and whole grains such as pasta, cereal and bread.

Pros and cons

Low in fat, grapefruit contains vitamins C and A, fibre, beta-carotenes and sodium. Phytochemicals in grapefruit are currently being researched for numerous health-promoting and disease-preventing properties. Some research even indicates there may be a link between the consumption of grapefruit and reduced insulin levels which curb hunger and facilitate weight loss, but this data is still preliminary.

Grapefruit, however, is low in protein, iron, calcium and several important vitamins and minerals, so this diet should be followed for a short period of time only. The restriction in calories may cause the dieter to suffer from fatigue, dizziness, nausea and constipation. Excessive consumption of caffeinated beverages may cause dehydration with loss of vital fluids from the body.

For successful weight loss to occur, the Grapefruit Diet must be strictly followed. No behavioural or lifestyle changes are suggested for the management of permanent weight loss, so it is extremely likely that the weight will be regained over time.

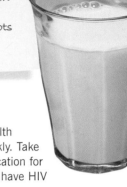

healthy tips
- Follow for 12 days only. Make sure that your plan includes a variety of fruits, vegetables and lots of water.

Is it for you?

Perfect for individuals in good health wanting to lose 4½kg (10lb) quickly. Take care if you are pregnant, on medication for diabetes or coronary problems, or have HIV or an AIDS-related condition.

Availability

All the foods in this diet can be purchased from any general food shop or supermarket.

Lifestyle changes

In general none but physical activity may be recommended, depending on the source used to obtain information about the diet.

of unsweetened grapefruit juice.

wednesday	thursday	friday
½ grapefruit or 120ml grapefruit juice (unsweetened), 2 eggs (any style), 2 slices bacon, black coffee or tea	½ grapefruit or 120ml grapefruit juice (unsweetened), 2 eggs (any style), 2 slices bacon, black coffee or tea	½ grapefruit or 120ml grapefruit juice (unsweetened), 2 eggs (any style), 2 slices bacon, black coffee or tea
½ grapefruit or 120ml grapefruit juice (unsweetened), meat or fish (any style or amount), salad with low-fat or no-fat dressing, black coffee or tea	½ grapefruit or 120ml grapefruit juice (unsweetened), meat or fish (any style or amount), salad with low-fat or no-fat dressing, black coffee or tea	½ grapefruit or 120ml grapefruit juice (unsweetened), meat or fish (any style or amount), salad with low-fat or no-fat dressing, black coffee or tea
½ grapefruit or 120ml grapefruit juice (unsweetened), meat or fish (any style, any amount), vegetables (any green, yellow or red vegetables cooked in butter or with any seasoning), black coffee or tea	½ grapefruit or 120ml grapefruit juice (unsweetened), meat or fish (any style, any amount), vegetables (any green, yellow or red vegetables cooked in butter or with any seasoning), black coffee or tea	½ grapefruit or 120ml grapefruit juice (unsweetened), meat or fish (any style, any amount), vegetables (any green, yellow or red vegetables cooked in butter or with any seasoning), black coffee or tea
1 glass tomato juice or 1 glass skimmed milk	1 glass tomato juice or 1 glass skimmed milk	1 glass tomato juice or 1 glass skimmed milk

Resources

www.grapefruit-diet.org

www.thinthin.com/article0160.html

Thompson, D.L., Ahrens, M.J. *The Grapefruit Solution* (2004, Linx Corp.)

LONG-TERM PLAN

FLEXIBILITY

FAMILY FRIENDLY

COST

STRENGTH OF SCIENCE

JUICING DIET

A variation on the fasting diet, this "drinking" plan includes only juices and teas.

Diet history
Unknown but there are several books by different authors available on it.

How does it work?
The juicing diet is a partial fast that includes some juices and broths. As a very low-calorie diet, it results in a state of ketosis from the breakdown of muscle and fat that is used up by the body as energy.

Juicing decreases some of the negative effects of a complete fast because it is not completely devoid of nutrients and includes carbohydrates that can be used as a source of energy, as well as vitamins and minerals. Carbohydrates are needed for blood glucose and the Juicing Diet provides a small amount of carbohydrate and calories. Consuming juices, water and broths partially minimizes dehydration and reduces the loss of potassium, sodium and other nutrients common in total fasting.

Many juicing diets encourage the preparation of raw juices with juicers and recommend specific drink concoctions for colonic cleansing. Although the Juicing Diet may be used for weight loss, it is often part of a cleansing ritual or a combination of both.

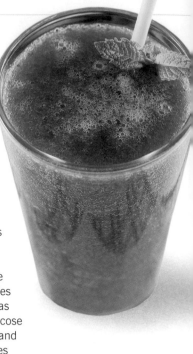

see also
fasting 126

sample menu This plan should only be

	day 1	day 2
snack 1	herb tea	herb tea
morning	juice, water	juice, water
snack 2	juice, water	juice, water
lunch	broth, water	broth, water
snack 3	juice, water	juice, water
supper	broth, water	broth, water
snack 4	juice or herb tea, water	juice or herb tea, water

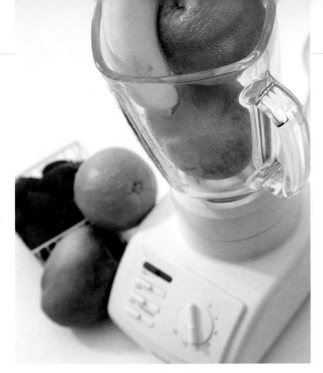

This diet should only be followed for a couple of days and the occurring weight loss will be the result of a combination of factors: low calorie intake, related water loss and a body fat reduction. Losing weight in this way long term can be dangerous.

Is it for you?
Juicing is likely to appeal to someone who wants an extremely low calorie diet but not the total – and more severe – full fast. It will suit those who enjoy drinking a lot of fluid and do not miss solid food or the act of chewing as part of their sit-down meal routine.

Juicing is a type of fast not generally recommended for all. Anyone with diabetes, heart-related and immuno-compromised (especially for the raw juicing plan) medical conditions should avoid this type of ritual at all costs.

Availability
All the fluids, juices and teas in this diet are readily available from any general food shop.

Many juicing diet books contain recipes for raw juices.

Pros and cons
Compared to a total fast, this diet does provide some carbohydrates, vitamins, minerals and calories which help to reduce several of the negative consequences related to muscle waste and the accumulation of cellular breakdown waste products in the bloodstream. It does not, however, completely succeed in the elimination of all the waste products produced.

Lifestyle changes
Usually none although walking and other mild forms of exercise are strongly recommended.

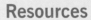

followed for a couple of days maximum.

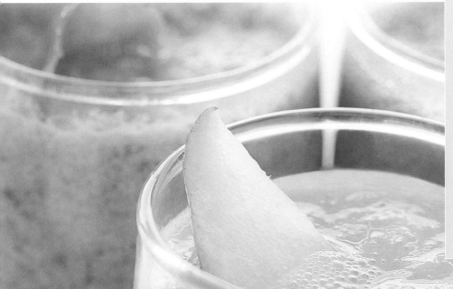

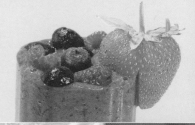

Resources

www.everydiet.org/liquid_diets.htm

Purcella, G., Cabot, S., Barry-Dee, C. *Juice Fasting Bible* (2007, Ulysses Press)

Airola, P. *How to Keep Slim, Healthy and Young with Juice Fasting* (1971, Health Plus Publishers)

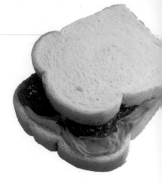

PEANUT BUTTER DIET

High-fibre monounsaturates in this eating plan will help you to feel full, but portion control is required.

LONG-TERM PLAN

FLEXIBILITY

FAMILY FRIENDLY

COST

STRENGTH OF SCIENCE

Diet history
Developed by writers from *Prevention Magazine*, parts of the diet first appeared in this publication. Holly McCord, a registered dietician and the magazine's nutrition editor, wrote a book shortly afterward.

How does it work?
A feeling of satisfaction and fullness, as well as variety, are important to diet adherence. The person dieting feels the satisfaction and sense of satiety associated with eating fats contained in a well-liked food prepared in a variety of ways. Thirty-five per cent of the diet's total measured caloric intake comes from "healthy" monounsaturated (16 per cent) and polyunsaturated (13 per cent) fats. Calories are limited through portion control.

Scientific findings indicate that replacing saturated fats (in some margarines, lard or coconut) with monounsaturated fats (in olive oil, rapeseed oil or nuts) is essential for maintaining a healthy heart.

In this diet, peanut butter provides most of the monounsaturated fats, but other nuts, avocados, rapeseed or olive oil can be used as well. About half of the total calories come from the carbohydrates in

healthy tips
- Plentiful sources of monounsaturated fats include olive oil, rapeseed oil, peanut oil, hazelnuts, avocados and peanuts.

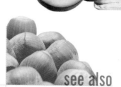

see also
volumetrics 108

sample menu
Peanut butter helps with satiety, but be mindful

	saturday	sunday	monday	tuesday
morning	220g grapefruit sections, mushroom omelette, 1 slice multigrain bread	25g puffed wheat cereal, ½ glass skimmed milk, 140g strawberries	100ml apple sauce, 2 tbsp peanut butter, 2 wholegrain waffles, ½ glass orange juice	1 banana, 100g orange sections, 100g bran flakes, ½ glass skimmed milk
lunch	salad (400g spinach, 2 tbsp peanuts, 2 tbsp raisins, 1 tsp oil and vinegar dressing), 1 slice multigrain bread, 1 tsp corn/rapeseed margarine	salad (200g cos, ½ cucumber, 75g carrots, 10 cherry tomatoes), plain croutons, 1 tsp oil and vinegar dressing	200g green salad with 1 tbsp oil vinegar dressing, 30g chicken breast sautéed in 1 tbsp corn oil, 170g asparagus, 120g grapes	salad (100g cos and iceberg, 30g low-fat mozzarella, 100g mixed dry-roasted nuts), 1 tsp oil and vinegar dressing, 1 wholewheat roll, grape juice and diet ginger ale
supper	55g grilled salmon, 180g green beans, 150g bulgur, 1 wholewheat roll, 300g salad (lettuce, tomatoes and carrots), 1 tsp oil and vinegar dressing	80g grilled tuna, 160g courgettes, 160g yellow squash, onions, 150g spinach salad, 1 tsp oil and vinegar dressing, 10 wholewheat crackers, 1½ tsp corn or rapeseed margarine, 225ml orange juice	75g wholewheat spaghetti, 50ml marinara sauce, 2 tbsp low-fat mozzarella, 180g green beans with 2 tsp corn oil margarine	80g baked ham, 200g Caesar salad, 2 tsp oil and vinegar dressing, 200g asparagus
snack 1	280g honeydew	3 sponge fingers, 70g blueberries	100g calorie-free jelly, 4 crackers, 2 tsp sugar-free jam	4 crackers, 2 tbsp peanut butter
snack 2	1 glass skimmed milk with 4 tsp peanut butter	100g soft vanilla frozen yogurt, 2 tbsp peanut butter	peanut butter shake with 2 tbsp peanut butter	celery and carrot sticks

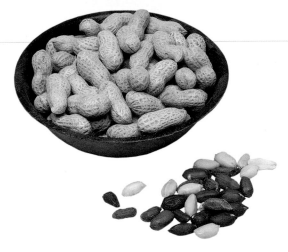

grains, vegetables, fruit and beans. Also included are a variety of foods from all the major food groups in a limited number of servings, sizes and portions. This includes three fruit servings, nine vegetable servings and two servings of calcium-rich foods (low-fat dairy and calcium-fortified orange juice). The daily peanut butter intake is limited to four tablespoons for women and six tablespoons for men as part of some prepared foods. The 28-day plan allows 1,500 calories a day (women) and 2,200 calories (men). The book offers recipes for a variety of peanut butter dishes and snacks such as peanut butter pudding, peanut butter ice cream shake, peanut butter hot chocolate and peanut butter ice cream.

Pros and cons

Scientific evidence supports the effectiveness of a calorie-controlled diet that includes variety, portion control, popular foods and satiety. The fats promote a healthier heart and are the recommended replacements for saturated fats but this is not an eating plan for life. Peanut butter is high in calories so it is important to control portion sizes, use level measures and observe the recipe amounts to stay within the planned low calorie intake or daily calorie limit. Some foods in the menu plans require careful preparation but simple recipes are also included.

Is it for you?

Ideal for lovers of peanut butter and people who enjoy whole grains. Avoid if you have difficulty swallowing, have extremely high blood triglycerides or are allergic to nuts.

Availability

Most foods in this diet can be bought from general food shops or supermarkets.

Lifestyle changes

The plan advises 45 minutes of physical activity staggered throughout the day rather than in one block. Muscle burns more calories than fat so there is emphasis on exercise that builds up muscle as well as reducing body fat, thus increasing the body's energy burning capacity.

treats

PICK FROM:
- biscuits
- spritzers
- low-fat cakes
- sugar-free jelly

of portion sizes to avoid excess calories.

wednesday	thursday	friday
1 glass orange juice, 75g porridge, 120ml skimmed milk, 2 tbsp peanut butter	160g apple slices, butter, 1 slice wholewheat toast, 1 tbsp peanut	110g grapefruit sections, 120ml apple sauce, 1 slice wholewheat bread, 2 tsp peanut butter
salad: 2 cups cos, 5 cherry tomatoes, 2 tbsp dry-roasted peanuts, 15g turkey breast, 1 tsp oil and vinegar dressing, 100ml skimmed milk	chalupa with beans, cheese, lettuce and tomato, green beans with 1 tsp corn oil margarine, 225ml orange juice	salad: 200g spinach, 150g beetroot, 50g orange sections, 15g dry-roasted pecans, 1 tsp oil and vinegar dressing
110g hummus, 1 wholewheat pitta bread, 150g tabouli, 200g spinach salad, 2 tsp oil and vinegar dressing, 1 glass tomato juice	80g grilled cod with 1 tsp corn oil, 75g diced redskin potatoes with 1 tsp olive oil, 150g beetroot, 200g salad: lettuce, tomatoes and carrots, 1 tsp oil and vinegar dressing	240ml vegetable soup, 200g green salad, 1 tsp oil and vinegar dressing, apple
100g orange sections	140g honeydew, 2 tbsp pecans	2 slices wholewheat bread, 2 tbsp peanut butter, ½ glass skimmed milk
140g watermelon	tall latte with skimmed milk, ½ wholewheat bagel, 1 tsp corn or rapeseed margarine	smoothie (½ banana with 100ml skimmed milk)

Resources

www.peanut-institute.org/index.html

McCord, H. *The Peanut Butter Diet* (2001, St. Martin's Paperbacks)

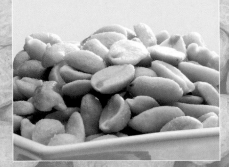

LONG-TERM PLAN

FLEXIBILITY

FAMILY FRIENDLY

COST

STRENGTH OF SCIENCE

THE ABS DIET

The Abs Diet promises a six-week plan to flatten your stomach and keep you lean for life.

Diet history
Published in 2004, *The Abs Diet* was written by David Zinczenko, Editor-in-Chief of *Men's Health* magazine. It appeared on the *New York Times* bestseller list.

How does it work?
The diet includes three meals and three snacks a day of about 1,900 calories. Although it is not as low in calories as some other diets, some of the calories are used up through the exercise regime that is part of the plan. Snacks should be eaten two hours before larger meals. According to the plan, all meals and snacks should contain at least two foods from the following list to supposedly increase natural fat burners and protect you from injury and illness:
- **A**lmonds and other nuts
- **B**eans and legumes
- **S**pinach and other green vegetables

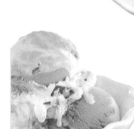

see also
atkins 42
south beach 64

sample menu
This plan emphasizes the recommended foods

	saturday	sunday	monday	tuesday
morning	Halle Berries Smoothie*	wholewheat pitta, low-fat cream cheese, 55g deli turkey or ham	Abs Diet Ultimate Power Smoothie*	scrambled egg sandwich, sliced tomato, 120ml orange juice
lunch	Chilli Con Turkey*	2 scrambled eggs, 2 slices wholegrain toast, 1 banana, 225ml skimmed milk	turkey sandwich on wholegrain bread, 225ml skimmed milk, apple	salad with cos, tomatoes, parmesan cheese, flaxseed, grilled chicken and fat-free Italian dressing
supper	Cheat Meal – whatever you want or crave	BBQ King*	Mas Macho Meatballs*	Bodacious Brazilian Chicken*
snack 1	1 bowl high-fibre cereal, 280g low-fat yogurt	2 tsp peanut butter, 1 can low-sodium V-8	2 tsp peanut butter, raw vegetables	2 tsp peanut butter, 1 bowl porridge
snack 2	3 slices deli roast beef, 1 orange	3 slices deli roast beef, 1 slice fat-free cheese	30g almonds, 150g berries	3 slices deli turkey, 1 orange
snack 3	Halle Berries Smoothie*	30g almonds, 80g low-fat ice cream	Abs Diet Ultimate Power Smoothie*	30g almonds, 110g cantaloupe

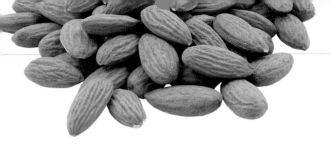

- **D**airy (fat-free or low-fat milk, yogurt or cheese)
- **I**nstant porridge (unsweetened, unflavoured)
- **E**ggs
- **T**urkey and other lean meats
- **P**eanut butter
- **O**live oil
- **W**holegrain breads and cereals
- **E**xtra-protein (whey) powder
- **R**aspberries and other berries

The diet limits refined carbohydrates, saturated fats, trans fats, alcohol and high-fructose corn syrup, and allows one meal a week when you can eat anything you want. It also includes optional exercise for the first two weeks and then a twenty-minute full body workout three days a week for weeks three to six.

Pros and cons
The diet is nutritionally sound in that it increases fruits, vegetables and whole grains while substituting healthy fats for saturated and trans fats. It does recommend a high protein intake of one gram per pound of body weight and claims that this extra protein will increase metabolic rate because of the thermic effect of food and its high satiety value. It includes an exercise regime that focuses on strength training, brisk walking and abdominal work.

Is it for you?
This plan will suit persons who are interested in losing belly fat and feeling better as they age. The high protein intake may be a problem for those with kidney disease, and there is some scientific evidence that high-protein diets may increase, not decrease, disease risk. Also, those with allergies to foods in the twelve food groups (such as nuts) should avoid this plan.

Availability
Most of the recommended foods are widely available in grocery shops and the whey protein powder is available in health-food shops.

Lifestyle changes
Exercise is an important part of the Abs Diet.

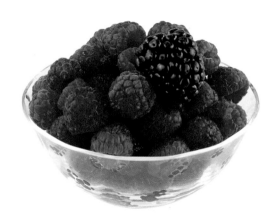

and one "cheat" meal per week.

wednesday	thursday	friday
Strawberry Field Marshall Smoothie*	wholegrain bread, 1 tsp peanut butter, All-Bran cereal, skimmed milk, 100g berries	Banana Split Smoothie*
tuna on ½ wholewheat roll	bacon and turkey BLT roll-up in wholewheat tortilla	tuna salad with wholewheat muffin
Chilli-Peppered Steak*	Philadelphia Fryers*	Chilli Con Turkey*
30g almonds, 30g raisins	230g low-fat yogurt, 1 can low-sodium V-8	30g almonds, 120g cantaloupe
1 stick of cheese, raw vegetables	3 slices deli roast beef, 1 orange	2 tsp peanut butter, 1 slice wholegrain bread
Strawberry Field Marshall Smoothie*	2 tsp peanut butter, 80g low-fat ice cream	Banana Split Smoothie*

Resources
www.TheAbsDiet.com

Zinczenko, D. *The Abs Diet* (2004, Rodale)

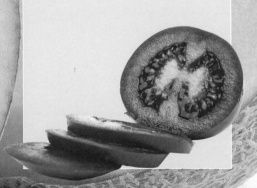

* Recipe in Zinczenko, D. *The Abs Diet*.

LONG-TERM PLAN

FLEXIBILITY

FAMILY FRIENDLY

COST

STRENGTH OF SCIENCE

BULL'S-EYE FOOD GUIDE

A quick-and-easy dietary system for selecting the healthiest foods possible, this eating programme organizes them into food groups based on the nutrients and chemicals they contain.

Diet history

Developed by Josephine Connolly Schoonen, MS, RD, at the Department of Family Medicine, State University of New York at Stony Brook, the *Bull's-Eye Food Guide* was published in 2004 as the result of the author's efforts in assisting patients with weight management. The guide is presented as a "journey" to improve eating style through empowerment and letting go of those habits associated with the consumption of excess calories. A three-ring target or "bull's-eye" categorizes foods according to different nutritional values, and this is divided into six groups.

How does it work?

Although structured differently from the USDA Food Guide, this new dietary system categorizes food according to its food group as well as its nutrient content, including vitamins, minerals, fibre, sugar, fat and sodium. It is still based on the scientific assumption that a combination of all the food groups promotes optimal health. There are also bull's-eye guides for low, moderate and high carbohydrate levels.

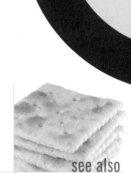

see also
fat is not your fate 100
volumetrics 108
rainbow 172

sample menu

This is one of the few plans that has water, a

	lower 1200	lower 1800	moderate 1200	moderate 1800
morning	2 slices light bread, 2 tsp peanut butter, 120ml 1% milk	2 slices light bread, 4 tsp peanut butter, 120ml 1% milk	40g cereal, 170g strawberries, 2 walnuts, 240ml 1% milk	50g cottage cheese, 75g blueberries, 10 crackers, 2 walnuts, 240ml 1% milk
lunch	lettuce, carrots, peppers, 70g chickpeas, 30g chicken, oil and vinegar, 100g melon, 100g low-fat yogurt	lettuce, carrots, peppers, 70g chickpeas, 55g chicken, oil and vinegar, 100g melon, 100g low-fat yogurt	broccoli frittata*, 50g tomatoes, 5 crackers	1 pitta bread, 2 hard-boiled eggs, 2 tsp mayonnaise, ½ tsp mustard, 175g beans, 125g watermelon
supper	80g turkey, 100g vegetables, 2 tsp olive oil and garlic, small baked potato	110g turkey, 200g vegetables, 2 tsp olive oil and garlic, medium-baked potato	55g pork with mustard dill sauce*, 75g carrots, 150g broccoli, 150g potatoes	tri-colour pasta and 225g prawns*, 200g broccoli
snack 1	smoothie with ½ banana, 240ml 1% milk	smoothie with ½ banana, 1 scoop soya protein powder, 240ml 1% milk	½ banana	200g low-fat yogurt, 2 dried apricots
snack 2	6 almonds	6 almonds	240ml 1% milk	150g wholegrain cereal squares, 6 almonds

Each of these guides is divided into six groups: grain, starch and sugar; milk and yogurt; fat; protein; fruit; and vegetable. The foods within each of the guide's rings are graphically presented by colour according to nutritional value. From the centre outwards, green is for "Go foods", yellow for "OK foods", and red for "Stop foods".

"Go foods" constitute the majority of the diet as they have the most nutritional value and may be eaten daily. "OK foods" are also healthy and can be eaten on a daily basis, but have less nutritional value. "Stop Foods" should be limited on a daily basis.

All guides include water at the centre, with eight or more glasses per day recommended. Individuals can make their preferred food choices and follow a structured eating plan with the best range of calories, carbohydrates, proteins and fats specific to their weight goals.

It is also suggested that weight-loss effort should be in stages of 7–9kg (15–20lb), followed by a gradual increase in food intake to maintain the loss for two to four weeks. These "maintenance breaks" should continue until the desired weight is achieved to optimize maintenance.

Pros and cons

The plan includes a variety of foods representing all the groups and provides individuals with a structured "road map" to healthy eating based on their needs and goals. It may be challenging for some to determine which guide is appropriate for their needs. Following the plan can be confusing due to the wide variety of choices.

Is it for you?

The Bull's-Eye Food Guide may suit those who prefer a highly structured plan or who are focusing on long-term change as they will like the breaks that allow for more permanent changes in eating habits. Anyone planning on following the low or high carbohydrate guides should consult a doctor and a registered dietician before embarking on the plan. This is especially important for children, adolescents, pregnant or breastfeeding women and the elderly.

Availability

All of the foods in the Bull's-Eye diet are widely available at any food shop.

Lifestyle changes

The daily consumption of water and regular physical activity are emphasized. Long-term lifestyle changes are integrated with the recommendation of "maintenance breaks" and behaviour is identified in relation to overeating.

key nutrient, at its core.

moderate 2400	high 1200	high 1800	Resources
3 slices bread, 4 tsp peanut butter, ½ banana, 240ml 1% milk	40g cereal, 75g blueberries, 240ml 1% milk	140g porridge, 1 peach, 240ml 1% milk	www.bulls-eyefoodguide.com

www.xenical.com/bulls_eye.asp |
lettuce, carrots, peppers, 140g chickpeas, 55g chicken, oil and vinegar, 5 crackers, 2 plums	lettuce, carrots, peppers, 70g chickpeas, 30g chicken, oil and vinegar, 1 orange	2 slices bread, 55g turkey, lettuce, ⅛ avocado, 75g carrots, 100g red pepper	Connolly Schoonen, J. *Losing Weight Permanently with the Bull's-Eye Food Guide* (2004, Bull Publishing Company)
140g chicken, 200g sautéed vegetables, 2 tsp olive oil, 300g potato, 6 cashews	55g chicken, 200g sautéed vegetables, 1 tsp olive oil, 1 medium potato	tofu stir-fry with broccoli, mushrooms, carrots and soya beans*	
protein smoothie: 120g strawberries, 1 scoop soya protein powder, 240ml 1% milk	smoothie: 170g strawberries, 240ml 1% milk	200g low-fat yogurt, 75g blueberries, 6 tbsp grape nut cereal	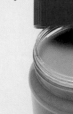
trail mix: 12 almonds, 150g wholegrain cereal squares, 2 tbsp raisins	5 wholewheat low-fat crackers	1 nectarine, 10 peanuts	

Notes: Use wholegrain breads, cereals, pasta and crackers, and brown rice.
   * Recipes from *Losing Weight Permanently with the Bull's-Eye Food Guide*.

LONG-TERM PLAN

FLEXIBILITY

FAMILY FRIENDLY

COST

STRENGTH OF SCIENCE

EAT, DRINK, AND WEIGH LESS

This plan uses a food pyramid that differs from other current popular pyramids such as the US MyPyramid and the Mediterranean Food Guide.

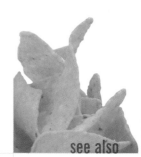

Diet history
This weight-loss book is co-authored by the well-known doctor and writer Walter Willett, from the Harvard School of Public Health, and cookery book author Mollie Katzen *(Moosewood Cookbook)*. *Eat, Drink, and Weigh Less* (2006) follows Willett's earlier book *Eat, Drink, and Be Healthy* (2001) which focused on general healthy eating, and also included menus and tips for lowering calories. The latest title is specifically written for weight loss.

How does it work?
Eat, Drink, and Weigh Less is a 21-day plan that uses a food pyramid that is a variation of the Mediterranean Food Guide. The pyramid has daily exercise and weight awareness as its base, and the next level includes fruits, vegetables, plant oils and whole grains. The level above that has nuts, tofu, legumes, fish, seafood, poultry and eggs; and the level above that is dairy and/or calcium plus vitamin D supplements. Then comes a multivitamin level, followed by the top levels of the pyramid, which indicate optional consumption, and include alcohol in moderation and dark chocolate.

see also
mayo 102
mediterranean 160

sample menu
This plan is based on the author's variation of

	saturday	sunday	monday	tuesday
morning	fruit platter, 200g low-fat cottage cheese, wholegrain toast, 1 tsp peanut butter	½ pink grapefruit, scrambled eggs with broccoli, 1 tsp sugar, coffee, low-fat milk	sliced strawberries, low-fat yogurt, 1 slice wholegrain toast, 1 tsp peanut butter, 2 tsp jam	wholegrain French Toast, 1 tsp maple syrup, blueberries, 1 tsp honey
lunch	vegetable broth with wheat berries, nachos, green salad, vinaigrette dressing	ethereal broccoli soup, Mediterranean-style French lentil salad, wholegrain salad, orange	spinach soup, ricotta egg salad, wholegrain crackers	cantaloupe, cottage cheese, 10 almonds, 1 tsp raisins, wholegrain toast
supper	Madras vegetable curry, baked tofu, 100g brown rice, spiced yogurt, toasted almonds, raisins, orange	100g wholegrain pasta, tomato sauce, chicken cutlet, broccoli, salad, balsamic dressing, cantaloupe	tomato soup, baked stuffed pepper, green salad, ranch dressing, orange meringue cookies	baked fish, apple-glazed acorn squash, braised greens, wholewheat orzo, pear
snack	chocolate banana cake	black bean dip, raw vegetables	trail mix	trail mix, 1 teaspoon chocolate chips

The less frequently recommended foods at the top layers include butter and butterfat, lean red meats and refined carbohydrates including soda bread, white potatoes, white bread, sweets etc. The authors identify nine turning points, or fundamental shifts, that can be made. There are two vegetable categories – the A list, which can be eaten freely; and the B list, which are slightly higher in carbohydrates and therefore limited to one or two servings per day. Similarly, fruits are lower in sugar than B-list fruits, which are higher in sugar and are limited to one serving per day. The plan does not forbid animal proteins but recommends emphasis on vegetable and lean animal proteins. Hydration, primarily through pure water, is encouraged. The plan includes a self-assessment questionnaire called a "Body Score Card" that is to be used to determine the status and goals. "Mindful" eating by understanding hunger, not skipping meals, eating breakfast and snacking strategically are emphasized.

Pros and cons
The meal plans contain a variety of foods, and the book has a range of recipes and a "tool kit", with strategies for eating out in a variety of settings, and a shopping guide.

The 9 turning points
1. Eat lots of vegetables and fruits
2. Say yes to good fats
3. Update your carbohydrate
4. Choose healthy proteins
5. Stay hydrated
6. Drink alcohol in moderation
7. Take a multivitamin daily
8. Move more
9. Eat mindfully all day long
(Katzen and Willett, 2006)

The diet includes some information about exercise and maintenance.

Is it for you?
This plan will appeal to those who want an approach to weight loss that focuses on healthy eating and gradual development of positive food behaviours and choices. People with special health conditions should consult a doctor prior to starting any weight-loss plan.

Availability
All foods can be bought in any general food shop.

Lifestyle changes
Start with 30 minutes' exercise a day, eat mindfully and use "what if" strategies.

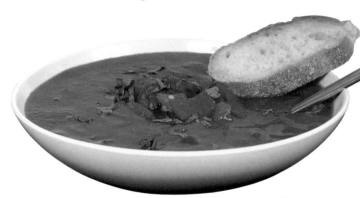

some other existing food pyramids.

wednesday	thursday	friday	**Resources**
raspberries, 100g wholegrain cereal, 110ml low-fat milk, 1 tsp sugar, coffee, low-fat milk	½ pink grapefruit, frittata with peas and goat's cheese, 1 tsp sugar, coffee, low-fat milk	cooked wholegrain cereal, 100ml low-fat milk, peach, 1 tsp sugar, coffee	www.eatdrinkandweighless.com Katzen, M., Willett, W. *Eat, Drink, and Weigh Less* (2006, Hyperion)
vegetable broth with egg, large mixed green salad with chickpeas, Balsamic dressing, orange	gazpacho, open-face cheese sandwich, mixed vegetables, buttermilk dressing, apple	mushroom barley vegetable broth, lean turkey burger, wholegrain bun, condiments, orange	
roasted chicken breast, courgettes, Parmesan cheese, marinated white beans, mixed grains, cashews, peach with yogurt	mushroom barley burger, tomato-based salsa, green beans, spaghetti squash, 110ml fruit sorbet	Miso soup with tofu, buckwheat noodles, cashews and greens, steamed chicken breast, marinated cucumbers, tangerines	
smoothie	170g yogurt-coated nuts	vegetables, salsa, 10 tortilla chips	

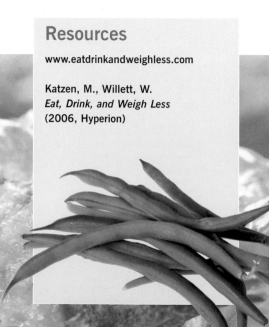

Note: Recipes, menus and amounts are in *Eat, Drink, and Weigh Less*.

LONG-TERM PLAN

FLEXIBILITY

FAMILY FRIENDLY

COST

STRENGTH OF SCIENCE

FAT IS NOT YOUR FATE DIET

This weight-loss programme is designed for people with genetic predispositions to obesity and/or chronic diseases. Based on the person's phenotype, the plan is designed to achieve healthy weight in an individual manner.

Diet history

In 1994, Dr Jeffrey M. Friedman identified the first obesity gene. He discovered that a genetic defect can affect the body's ability to use nutrients adequately and that this may contribute to obesity – a concept known as nutrigenomics. It describes how balanced nutrition can help overcome side-effects caused by a genetic predisposition to obesity, "that will allow you to outsmart your genes and beat them at their own game." Fat is Not Your Fate provides detailed examples from clinical cases in which dieters followed an evidence-based diet suited to their phenotype with excellent results.

Sun-dried tomatoes.

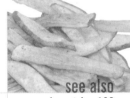

see also
volumetrics 108

sample menu
Determine your phenotype, then follow the

	phenotype H	phenotype A	phenotype B	phenotype C
morning	multigrain cereal with flaxseed and soya milk, dried red cherries, maple syrup, green tea	poached egg, sliced French baguette with Swiss cheese, pineapple juice	lemon squeezer smoothie (banana, raspberries, vanilla frozen yogurt, lemon sorbet), wheat bread with margarine	soya sausage, buckwheat pancakes with fresh blueberries, hot tea
lunch	roast pork fillet steak, mushroom risotto, sautéed spinach, lemon-infused water	roast turkey sandwich, oatmeal bread, tomato, lettuce, avocado and baby carrots, water	carrot chowder with turkey, raisin bread, mixed vegetables, decaf coffee	grilled chicken breast, brown rice, roasted Sicilian vegetables, non-caloric drink
supper	bean chilli, corn bread, mixed green salad, non-caloric orange drink	wholegrain flour tortilla, kidney beans, yellow corn, shredded cheddar cheese, spring salad, apple juice	garlic chicken with goat's cheese, baked sweet potato, zesty green beans, green tea	grilled fresh tuna, green salad with olives, rye bread with margarine, red grapes, lime water
snack	tangerine, tea	multigrain Cheerios with 1% fat soya milk	popcorn, lime-flavoured water	dried cherries, sparkling water

How does it work?

Nutrigenomics is a new concept and its popularity is fast emerging. To follow this diet, the dieter must know his or her genetic predisposition or phenotype. They are as follows: Phenotype A (weight gain linked to addiction); Phenotype B (weight gain linked with high blood pressure); Phenotype C (weight gain linked to cardiovascular disease); Phenotype D (weight gain linked to diabetes); Phenotype E (weight gain linked to emotional eating); and Phenotype H (weight gain linked to hormones). The book provides a self-assessment questionnaire to determine the individual's phenotype, negative triggers to weight gain and alternatives to replace those negative prompts.

The diet should be followed for at least 12 weeks and involves keeping food intake records up to date. In the first two weeks, the dieter can go on a fast-track diet that eliminates "sweets, treats and alcohol" in order to provide quick weight loss and give a person the necessary motivation to then follow the phenotype diet.

Pros and cons

The self-assessment of phenotype, food habits and recognizing overeating triggers increases a person's awareness of their individual habits and conditions, and provides the motivation to make healthier choices. The Fat is Not Your Fate Diet uses the hand (fist, palm and thumb) to measure out portion sizes, detailed food lists, and quick and simple or more complex sample menus. The hand technique is an easy way of measuring the amount of food eaten. The sample menus include culture-specific items that broaden the suitability of the diet.

Also, the plan provides menu samples for both men and women. The programme's success depends on the dieter's commitment to keep food records, perform self-assessments and learn about food portions.

Is it for you?
The diet is suitable for most adults.

Availability
Most the foods in this diet are readily available from a large supermarket.

Lifestyle changes
During the first two weeks, a fast-track phase can be followed, if desired, during which the dieter avoids alcohol, sweets and treats. These foods will be gradually re-introduced to the phenotype diet. Fat is Not Your Fate introduces exotic and uncommon fruit and vegetables in order to increase variety.

appropriate programme.

phenotype D	phenotype E (6 mini meals)
porridge with 1% soya milk, pink grapefruit, coffee	toasted almond muesli with raisins and ground flaxseed meal, low-fat soya milk, green tea
lentil-vegetable soup, mozzarella cheese, pumpernickel, green beans, non-caloric drink	vegetable and cheese pizza, green salad with nuts, flavoured water
mozzarella and spinach pasta, spiced carrot-raisin salad, seven-grain roll, low-fat margarine, mango tea	polenta topped with parmesan cheese, diced tomatoes, spinach, unsweetened orange juice
dried cranberry and walnut mix	cheddar cheese with low-fat wheat crackers, lime-flavoured water
	cappucino, soya milk, wholegrain Lavash
	vanilla yogurt, fresh pear

Resources

www.fatisnotyourfate.com

www.dnadiet.org

Mitchell, S., Christie, C., *Fat is Not Your Fate: Outsmart Your Genes and Lose Weight Forever* (2006, Simon & Schuster)

LONG-TERM PLAN

FLEXIBILITY

FAMILY FRIENDLY

COST

STRENGTH OF SCIENCE

MAYO CLINIC HEALTHY WEIGHT PROGRAM

A plan based on assessing one's readiness to diet, fitness levels, identifying weight and daily calorie goals, and suitable daily food-group serving recommendations.

Diet history

The Mayo Clinic is a comprehensive healthcare system that provides medical nutrition therapy – including weight-loss counselling – as one of its services. A mythical diet of unknown origin, the so-called Mayo Clinic Diet (also called a grapefruit diet) became popular and recently resurfaced as the New Mayo Clinic Diet. It promotes grapefruit, eggs or meat for quick weight loss but is not affiliated with the Mayo Clinic. A recent book, *The Mayo Clinic Healthy Weight Program* (2006), was probably published to counteract this diet myth and help promote a science-based approach to health and weight management. The Mayo Clinic Healthy Weight Program is the only plan affiliated to the clinic.

How does it work?

The plan individually assesses a person's readiness to diet, establishes weight goals, identifies calorie limits, and uses a plan based on food groups and corresponding serving sizes. It was designed to work around the basic formula that, in order to lose ½kg (1lb) of fat, the

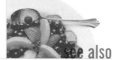

see also
weight watchers 80
bull's-eye 96
mypyramid 162

sample menu

A well-planned 1,500-calorie menu, such as

	saturday	sunday	monday	tuesday
morning	120ml pineapple juice, 1 egg, 50g polenta, coffee or tea	120ml orange juice, 1 muffin, 2 plums, coffee or tea	120ml apple juice, 55g spoon-size shredded wheat, ½ bagel, fat-free cream cheese, coffee or tea	120ml orange juice, 100g porridge, coffee or tea
lunch	salad: 50g kasha, 100g cauliflower, 75g mushrooms, and diced pepper, 1 apple, calorie-free drink	baked pork loin, ½ medium baked potato, 75g green beans, cucumber slices, 3 dates, calorie-free drink	2 slices wholegrain bread, 1 veggie burger, 100g spinach, 8 cherry tomatoes, fat-free dressing, 1 orange, calorie-free drink	1 muffin, half-fat mozzarella, 120ml pizza sauce, 70g carrot sticks, 1 kiwi fruit, calorie-free drink
supper	2 slices sourdough bread, lentil soup, 100g shredded cabbage, 1 peach, calorie-free drink	egg-substitute omelette, 50g orzo, 100g summer squash, 100g courgettes, 1 orange, calorie-free drink	grilled salmon, 100g rice, 100g asparagus, 80g beetroot, 1 banana, calorie-free drink	roasted turkey breast, 3 baby red potatoes, 100g broccoli, 100g cauliflower, 1 bell pepper, 1 peach, calorie-free drink
snack 1	120ml salsa, 10 baked crisps, calorie-free drink	200g plain popcorn, calorie-free drink	1 breadstick, 120ml vegetable juice	1 small muffin, 100g mixed berries
snack 2	1 frozen juice bar, 6 crackers, calorie-free drink	80ml vegetable soup, 6 wheat crackers, calorie-free drink	200g strawberries, sliced almonds, calorie-free drink	6 wheat crackers, calorie-free drink

weigh this up...
- You can substitute foods not on the list but ensure that the calorie, protein and fat content are similar to those of foods from the same group.

body must burn an additional 3,500 calories over the number of calories consumed.

The plan recommends taking small steps, losing no more than ½–1kg (1–2lb) a week, emphasizing positives, setting priorities, avoiding gimmicks, seeking support networks and concentrating on slow but steady weight loss.

Calorie levels are prescribed by weight and gender. Recommendations are given for every food group and calorie level in terms of number of servings and the size of portions. Lists of recommended vegetables, fruit, carbohydrates, protein, dairy, fats and sweets are included in the book. Although no specific foods are identified as "forbidden", each listed group has different calorie levels.

Pros and cons

The evidence supporting the Mayo Clinic Healthy Weight Program is strong. The diet uses a moderate approach to weight loss based on self-awareness, behavioural change, portion control and long-term commitment.

This dieting method will not appeal to those who want a short-term, quick-fix weight-loss plan. Moreover, the unlimited amount of fruit servings must be monitored with care to ensure the person dieting does not exceed his or her calorie goals by drinking too much fruit juice.

Is it for you?

This plan will appeal to those who like a holistic approach to weight loss that integrates wellness, physical activity and eating.

Availability

The foods in this diet can be readily bought from larger food shops. Some of the menu items need to be prepared according to the different recipe specifications but the number of calories for a given item are specified giving the dieter the freedom to substitute a similar item containing the same amount of calories.

Lifestyle changes

The plan requires a commitment to behavioural change and includes a fitness level assessment as well as physical activity recommendations.

free foods
- calorie-free foods or those with less than 20 calories per serving

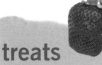

treats
PICK FROM:
- foods up to 75 calories
- angel cake
- jelly
- nuts

healthy tips
- Vegetables that are 25 calories or less per serving are: red or green peppers, green beans, cabbage and courgettes.

this one, can provide plenty of healthy foods.

wednesday	thursday	friday
120ml pineapple juice, 2 small pancakes, coffee or tea	120ml grapefruit juice, 55g wholegrain cereal, 1 glass skimmed milk, coffee or tea	120ml cranberry juice, 3 prunes, 2 slices wholewheat toast, coffee or tea
salad: 70g chickpeas, 200g spinach, 8 cherry tomatoes, 100g sliced cucumber, 1 breadstick, 1 kiwi fruit, calorie-free drink	roast chicken, 100g rice, 140g steamed kale, 100g water chestnuts, 1 nectarine, calorie-free drink	50g pasta, 25ml tomato sauce, shredded mozzarella, 100g broccoli, 1 pear, calorie-free drink
grilled prawns, 1 small roll, 75g baby carrots, 100g peas, 200g aubergine, 2 plums, calorie-free drink	100g pasta, 120ml marinara sauce, 100g summer squash, 1 breadstick, 1 banana, calorie-free drink	lean minced beef, 140g macaroni with tomato sauce, 1 tomato, 200g courgettes, 1 banana, calorie-free drink
1 nectarine, calorie-free drink	6 wheat crackers, 120ml vegetable juice	1 orange, calorie-free drink
14 small cheese crackers, calorie-free drink	1 tangerine, calorie-free drink	200g plain popcorn, calorie-free drink

Resources

www.mayoclinic.com/health/mayo-clinic-diet-book/GA00037

The Mayo Clinic Plan: 10 Essential Steps to a Better Body and Healthier Life (2006, Time)

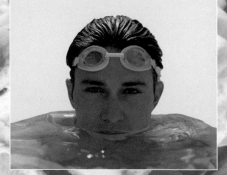

LONG-TERM PLAN

FLEXIBILITY

FAMILY FRIENDLY

COST

STRENGTH OF SCIENCE
●●

SONOMA DIET

Based on the laidback lifestyle and food of California's wine country, this Mediterranean-type eating guide favours low-calorie, healthy heart "power" foods.

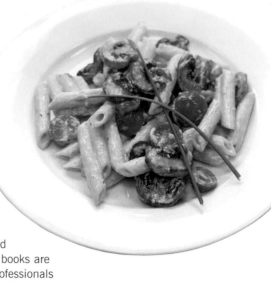

Diet history

The Sonoma Diet was devised by Connie Peraglie Guttersen, a registered dietician, gourmet chef and nutrition consultant at the Culinary Institute of America at Greystone, California. The first diet book was published in 2005 and followed by *The Sonoma Diet Cookbook* (2006). Both books are popular and often recommended by health professionals looking to promote a Mediterranean style of eating.

How does it work?

This meal plan encourages long-term weight loss through a healthy dietary guide that includes the Mediterranean staples of fruit, vegetables, fish, cheese, olive oil, nuts and wine. Based on 10 "power" foods (almonds, peppers, blueberries, broccoli, grapes, olive oil, spinach, strawberries, tomatoes and whole grains), the rationale is

see also
mediterranean 160

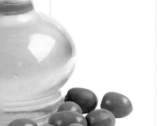

sample menu
The Sonoma Diet is a Mediterranean-type diet

	saturday	sunday	monday	tuesday
morning	2 slices wholewheat bread, 1 tbsp peanut butter	wholegrain cereal, milk	110g wholegrain cereal, 240ml skimmed milk	porridge, milk
lunch	greens with beans and artichoke hearts*, 75g raspberries	chicken and black bean wrap*, fresh fruit	black bean soup*, spinach salad with vinaigrette, 100g fresh berries	Sonoma salad with tomatoes and feta*, fresh fruit, 4 crackers
supper	Moroccan pork kebabs*, Tunisian carrot salad*, steamed brown rice, 1 glass pinot noir (optional)	wild mushroom barley risotto*, salad with lemon vinaigrette*, 1 glass merlot (optional)	pork tenderloin*, quinoa pilaf*, roasted courgette, 50g cantaloupe, 1 glass zinfandel (optional)	prawns with serranos*, grain medley*, 1 cup salad vinaigrette*, fruit, 1 glass sauvignon blanc (optional)
snack for men	100g broccoli, 3 soft cheese wedges, 75g blueberries, fat-free yogurt	2 sticks celery, 2 tbsp peanut butter, 1 stick of cheese, 150g baby carrots, 33 almonds	2 mozzarella cheese sticks, 2 sticks celery with 2 tbsp peanut butter, 33 almonds	150g baby carrots, 3 soft cheese wedges, 33 almonds
snack for women	100g broccoli, 1 soft cheese wedge, 50g blueberries, fat-free yogurt	2 sticks celery, 1 tbsp peanut butter, string cheese, 150g baby carrots, 11 almonds	2 sticks celery with 2 tbsp peanut butter, 22 almonds	150g baby carrots, 22 almonds

that the high nutrient density of these foods is evidence of their ability to protect against heart disease and other serious illnesses. The main emphasis of the Sonoma Diet is on unprocessed foods and what you *can* eat rather than on "forbidden" food lists.

The book includes three waves: Wave One lasts for up to 10 days and restricts some fruit and vegetables; Wave Two lasts for as long as is necessary to lose the desired weight; and Wave Three starts on the day that the target weight is reached.

Pros and cons

The abundance of fruit, vegetables and whole grains undoutedly makes the Sonoma Diet a healthy option and this corresponds to other science-based recommendations for healthy eating such as the Food Guide Pyramid.

Dieters who are not used to eating a lot of fruit and vegetables will find this plan a departure from what they know, and may also find it expensive. Eating more fruit and vegetables will not increase cost if balanced by a reduction of more costly meats and processed foods.

Is it for you?

Aimed at people who enjoy food, wine or simply want an eating and weight-maintenance lifetime plan, the Sonoma Diet is not designed to bring on a quick weight loss but is a lifelong programme that results in a gradual and steady drop. Depending on the current intake of processed,

energy-dense foods, it may not suit those who rely on these kinds of products and are not ready to commit to long-term changes in the foods that are normally eaten.

Availability

All the foods in this diet can be readily bought from any grocery shop or general supermarket.

Lifestyle changes

This lifestyle plan recommends exercise and behaviour management techniques, having regular meals, keeping a food and exercise diary, identifying and managing food-related cues to avoid overeating, plus dealing with stress and drawing up a plan for handling setbacks.

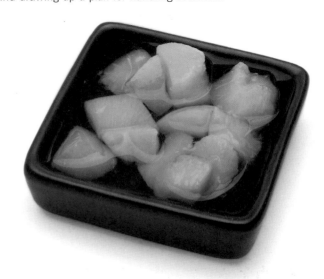

but includes foods from many cultures.

wednesday	thursday	friday
2 eggs, 1 slice wholewheat toast, 1 tbsp peanut butter	2 slices wholewheat toast, 1 tbsp peanut butter	ranchero omelet*
Sonoma express wrap*, grain medley*, fresh fruit	California chicken salad*, 1 wholegrain pitta	mixed greens with turkey and blue cheese*, 4 crackers
pork tenderloin*, spinach with vinaigrette*, fresh fruit, 1 glass cabernet (optional)	lentil soup*, fish with courgette relish*, 100ml salad vinaigrette*, 1 glass sauvignon blanc (optional)	chilli ginger beef and Asian vegetable medley*, fresh fruit, 1 glass rosé (optional)
2 tbsp yogurt cucumber sauce*, ½ wholewheat pitta, 100g raw courgettes, 22 almonds	fat-free yogurt, 100g strawberries, 2 soft cheese wedges, pepper strips, 22 almonds	25g hummus*, wholewheat pitta, cucumber slices, 2 sticks celery with 2 tbsp peanut butter
2 tbsp yogurt cucumber sauce*, ½ wholewheat pitta	2 tbsp yogurt cucumber sauce*, ½ wholewheat pitta, pepper strips	25g hummus*, wholewheat pitta, cucumber slices

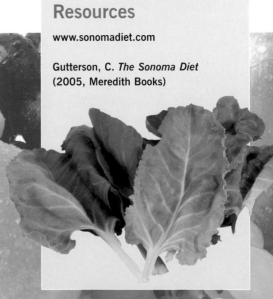

Resources

www.sonomadiet.com

Gutterson, C. *The Sonoma Diet* (2005, Meredith Books)

*Recipes included in Guttersen, C. *The Sonoma Diet*.

LONG-TERM PLAN

FLEXIBILITY

FAMILY FRIENDLY

COST

STRENGTH OF SCIENCE

TRI-COLOR DIET

Designed to produce permanent weight loss and add years of healthier living to your life, this colourful plan focuses on the intake of red, yellow, orange and green phytochemicals.

Diet history

Developed by Martin Katahn, founder and director of the Vanderbilt Weight Management Program and Professor of Psychiatry Emeritus at Vanderbilt University, the Tri-Color Diet was introduced in 1996. He is also well known for *The 200-Calorie Solution (1984)*, *Beyond Diet (1984)*, *The Rotation Diet (1987)*, *One Meal at a Time (1997)*, *The T-Factor Diet (2001)* and others.

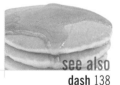

Increase colour and phytochemical intake by adding vegetables and herbs to soups and sandwiches.

How does it work?

This eating guide promises permanent weight management, no feelings of deprivation, and a lifelong strategy for the prevention of cancer, heart disease and other debilitating, age-related diseases.

Based on the inclusion of colourful phytochemicals present in plant food, the programme groups them into three categories: red, yellow/

see also
dash 138

sample menu

For easy menu planning, select a range of

	saturday	sunday	monday	tuesday
morning	fruit juice, cold cereal, fresh or dried fruit, wholegrain bread, drink	fresh fruit or juice, pancakes with maple syrup, drink	fruit juice, cold cereal, fresh or dried fruit, wholegrain bread, drink	fresh fruit or juice, French toast with maple syrup, drink
lunch	pasta/vegetable salad, roll or wholegrain bread, fruit drink	fruit or vegetable juice, poultry, cooked vegetable drink	fruit or vegetable juice, sandwich, vegetable side dish, fruit, drink	soup, sandwich with vegetable garnish, fruit, drink
supper	poultry, 2 vegetable side dishes, wholegrain bread, choice of fruit dessert	fish, cooked vegetable, small salad, wholegrain bread, choice of fruit dessert	fruit appetizer, main course from book recipes, side vegetable or salad, dessert recipe from book	fish, 2 vegetable side dishes, wholegrain bread, choice of fruit dessert
snack 1	fruit	fruit	fruit	fruit
snack 2	wholegrain	wholegrain	wholegrain	wholegrain

orange and green. Weight loss can be slowly obtained by following the diet's disease-prevention guidelines or more quickly using the Express Plan, which also emphasizes the incorporation of those nutritional principles that will need to be followed forever.

The ultimate goal is nine servings of fruit and vegetables a day and six to eleven grain servings with no more than 20 per cent of calories derived from fat. No foods are considered "bad" although some are limited, including fat (1 to 2 tablespoons per day, no more than 20 per cent of the total calories), red meat (once a week, ideally once a month, or never), fish and poultry (170g per day), primarily low-fat dairy products, no soft drinks (including diet soft drinks), and coffee intake limited to two cups a day. Suggestions for ethnic choices that fit the plan are also included.

Pros and cons

The increased intake of fruit, vegetables and whole grains is a positive approach to diet strongly supported by the scientific evidence on promoting health and weight loss.

Some dieters may find keeping to the recommended changes quite challenging in the long term especially if these are vastly different or poles apart from their current dietary habits. The programme advises starting with one recipe, one meal, one day at a time to gradually introduce the magnitude of the change. While this may appeal to those looking for a lifestyle change, it may be too dedicated and slow for others wanting immediate and

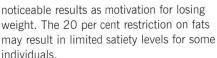

weigh this up...
• What is a phytochemical? Any chemical or nutrient that has biological activity in the body and is derived from a plant source.

noticeable results as motivation for losing weight. The 20 per cent restriction on fats may result in limited satiety levels for some individuals.

Is it for you?

The strong emphasis on natural plant-based foods could prove popular either with individuals wanting to avoid or cut down on meat consumption or with people interested in changing their dietary habits to reduce health risks. Anyone with kidney disease will not be able to consume all of the fruit and vegetables due to potassium restriction.

Availability

The foods in this diet are widely available and affordable.

Lifestyle changes

Physical activity, stress management and reducing environmental health risks are all integrated into the plan.

colours, which will also provide nutrient variety.

wednesday	thursday	friday	**Resources**
fresh fruit or juice, hot cereal with dried fruit, drink	fruit, leftover soup, wholegrain bread, drink	fruit or juice, leftover plant-food dish from dinner, wholegrain bread, drink	www2.wwnorton.com/catalog/ spring96/003920.htm
large salad, wholegrain bread or roll, fruit, drink	fruit or vegetable juice, fish, small salad, drink	soup, small luncheon salad, fruit, drink	Katahn, M. *The Tri-Color Diet* (1996, W. W. Norton & Co.)
poultry, cooked vegetables, small salad, wholegrain bread, choice of fruit dessert	3 or more plant-based dishes, wholegrain bread or roll, choice of fruit dessert	fruit appetizer, main course from book recipes, side vegetable or salad, dessert recipe from book	
fruit	fruit	fruit	
wholegrain	wholegrain	wholegrain	

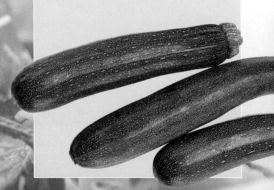

Note: The book offers generic meal plans rather than specific menus.

LONG-TERM PLAN
●●●

FLEXIBILITY
●●

FAMILY FRIENDLY
●●●

COST
●

STRENGTH OF SCIENCE
●●●

THE VOLUMETRICS WEIGHT-CONTROL PLAN

Feel full on fewer calories. *The Volumetrics Weight-Control Plan* is a diet book based on the principles of eating to increase satiety (satisfaction and fullness after eating).

Diet history

In addition to the above title, there is a subsequent book, *The Volumetrics Eating Plan* by Barbara Rolls, PhD (holder of the endowed Guthrie Chair of Nutritional Sciences at Pennsylvania State University) and Robert A. Barnett (award-winning food and nutrition journalist). The books are well known and are often recommended by health professionals because of their strong scientific basis and easy-to-use style.

How does it work?

Food choices are based on energy (calorie) density. Fat, fibre, protein and water content of foods all affect energy (calorie) density. By eating predominantly filling, low energy (calorie) dense foods, calories are controlled, smaller portions of a few high energy dense foods can be eaten, and the person will still lose weight. Examples of foods with low

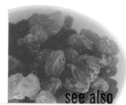

see also
bull's-eye 96
fat is not your fate 100

sample menu

Menus include nutrient-dense, high-fibre, low-

	saturday	sunday	monday	tuesday
morning	100g shredded wheat, 240ml skimmed milk	200g low-fat vanilla yogurt, 2 slices wholewheat toast, ½ tbsp light margarine, 240ml skimmed milk	50g raisin bran, 1 peach, 240ml skimmed milk	1 wholewheat muffin, 1 tbsp reduced-fat peanut butter, 240ml skimmed milk
lunch	140g bean and cheese burrito, 50ml salsa	turkey sandwich on 15cm wheat sub roll, 480ml vegetable soup	1 reduced-calorie entrée, salad, 60ml fat-free dressing	grilled chicken sandwich (no mayo), vegetables
supper	1 pitta pizza margherita, salad, 50ml fat-free dressing	80g poached salmon, salad, 60ml fat-free dressing, 1 wholewheat roll	75g wholewheat pasta, 150g mixed vegetables, 120ml prepared pasta sauce, 1 tbsp parmesan, 1 square of chocolate	stir-fried beef and mange-tout, 100g brown rice, 2 fortune cookies
snack 1	1 banana	40g low-fat vanilla ice cream	180ml cup broth, 4 fat-free cheese crackers	225g peaches in light syrup, 110g low-fat cottage cheese
snack 2	80g frozen fruit and juice bar	170g grapes	140g strawberries	1 pear

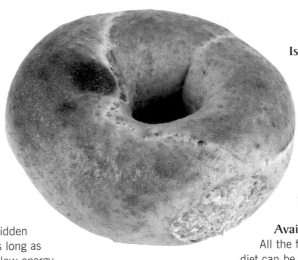

energy density include fruits and vegetables, skimmed milk, broth-based soups, fat-free salad dressings, pasta, cooked high-fibre grains, potatoes, legumes, low-fat meats, salads, low-fat soups, low-fat cheeses, cottage cheese, frozen yogurt and non-calorie drinks. The diet is complemented by regular exercise and behaviour management. There are no forbidden foods, and treats are allowed as long as the predominant eating style is low energy (calorie) density.

Is it for you?

It is not designed to produce quick weight loss. It is a lifestyle programme that results in slow and steady weight loss. It may require major changes to current eating patterns, depending on the person's intake of energy dense foods.

Availability

All the foods recommended in this diet can be bought in any grocery shop or supermarket.

Pros and cons

The diet is rich in nutrient-dense, but not calorie-dense, foods such as fruits and vegetables, which makes it healthy and corresponds to other science-based recommendations. Choosing low energy dense foods may be difficult to consistently maintain over time because of the prevalence of high energy dense foods, especially at parties, holidays and other social situations that involve eating.

Lifestyle changes

The authors state that "this is a lifestyle plan, not a diet". Recommended life-changing strategies include regular exercise and behaviour management techniques such as not skipping meals, keeping a food and exercise diary, identifying and managing cues to overeating, learning stress management and making a plan to handle setbacks.

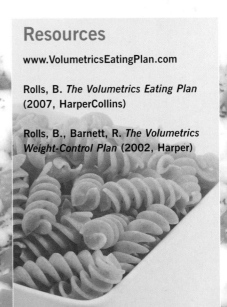

calorie foods to promote a healthy lifestyle change.

wednesday	thursday	friday
75g Cheerios, 40g dried apricots, 240ml skimmed milk	2 scrambled eggs, 2 tbsp salsa, 2 slices wholewheat toast, ½ tbsp light margarine, 240ml skimmed milk	100g bran flakes, 100g blueberries, 240ml skimmed milk
ham sandwich on 15cm wheat sub roll, 1 slice cheese, vegetables	1 tin broth, 1 wholewheat bagel, 1 tbsp reduced-fat peanut butter	1 small cheeseburger (no mayo), garden salad, 50ml fat-free dressing
80g baked pork chop, 200g wild rice, 125g broccoli (with lemon), 1 tbsp cheddar	1 reduced-calorie entrée, salad, 50ml fat-free dressing	80g baked chicken, 100g yellow rice, cucumber and dill salad
1 snack cup non-fat chocolate pudding	200g sugar-free, low-fat fruit yogurt	100g fruit sorbet
½ grapefruit	125g raspberries	1 apple

Resources

www.VolumetricsEatingPlan.com

Rolls, B. *The Volumetrics Eating Plan* (2007, HarperCollins)

Rolls, B., Barnett, R. *The Volumetrics Weight-Control Plan* (2002, Harper)

LONG-TERM PLAN

FLEXIBILITY

FAMILY FRIENDLY

COST

STRENGTH OF SCIENCE

3-HOUR DIET

This diet keeps hunger at bay by allowing you to eat at regular three-hour intervals.

Diet history

The plan was developed by fitness trainer Jorge Cruise who wrote the *8 Minutes in the Morning*® books on fitness and short workout routines. The 3-Hour Diet was developed in response to requests for a weight-loss plan that required little or no exercise and used techniques and concepts common to many other diets.

How does it work?

The plan revolves around the theory that timing mealtimes with precision – and not the elimination of carbohydrates – is crucial to successful weight control and includes a 3-Hour Timeline™ and 3-Hour Plate™. According to the timeline's rationale, eating every three hours avoids hunger pangs and the activation of the starvation protection mechanism (SPM), the thermic effect of food (using up calories for digestion) is maximized and blood glucose levels remain constant. There is no need for food restrictions or limitations on carbohydrate intake, and Visual Timing™ develops an automatic eating schedule that increases your awareness of when and how to eat.

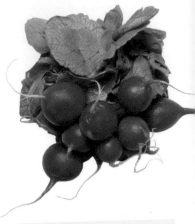

healthy tips
- Good sources of Omega fats include flax and salmon (Omega-3), soya bean oil and corn oil (Omega-6), olives, avocados and nuts (Omega-9).

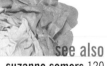

see also
suzanne somers 120

sample menu
Each meal should be about 400 calories and

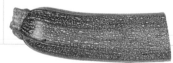

	saturday	sunday	monday	tuesday
morning	porridge, 1% milk, 50g dried cranberries	wheat flakes cereal, 2 tbsp sliced almonds, 1% milk, plum	egg-white omelette with cheese, 2 slices toast, 1 tsp margarine, fruit salad	low-fat muesli cereal, ½ banana, 1% milk, peach
lunch	plain burger, side salad, low-fat ranch dressing, 1 glass orange juice	honey-glazed ham, steamed carrots, side salad, Italian dressing, orange	grilled chicken breast, 225ml vegetable soup, roll	cheeseburger, side salad, 1 tsp low-fat dressing
supper	grilled chicken breast, baked potato, 1 tbsp rapeseed oil, mange-tout	grilled tuna, stewed tomatoes, artichoke hearts, 1 tbsp olive oil, couscous pilaf	soya burger, mushrooms, rice pilaf, greens, salad	grilled fish, spring greens with flax oil, cornbread
snack 1	100g sorbet	yogurt (100 calories)	biscuit pack (100 calories)	15g pretzels
snack 2	100g jelly	biscuit pack (100 calories)	15g baked tortilla chips	yogurt (100 calories)
snack 3	lettuce salad, 15 raisins, no-calorie dressing	1 rice cake, 1 tbsp fat-free cream cheese	6 almonds, jicama sticks, green tea	15g fruit pastels, apple

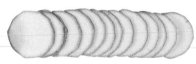

The 3-Hour Plate™ includes five to six portion-controlled daily eating "events" every three hours during this 28-day low-calorie food plan. The key to the diet are three square meals (about 400 calories each), two snacks (about 100 calories each) and one treat (up to 50 calories) for a total of 1,450 calories.

While carbohydrates are permitted, whole grains are promoted as "extra credit". Protein foods low in saturated fats (egg whites, white meat, low-fat yogurt, 1% milk) and foods rich in Omega-3 and Omega-9 fats are firm favourites. Red meat is also allowed.

Regular eating habits help to minimize low blood sugar levels and boost metabolism. You can either follow the book's pre-prepared meal plans or the dietary concepts based around customized meals.

Pros and cons

This structured, low-calorie eating plan with its small frequent mealtimes and numerous strategies encourages compliance in the dieter by taking even favourite foods and dining out into consideration. You can eat whatever you like so long as it is within the recommended timeframe and caloric allowance. Although the diet's weight-loss claim is an average of 1kg (2lb) per week, this will ultimately depend on an individual's constitution. The plan's wordy terminology with its new trademarked terms for well-known dieting strategies or techniques could initially be perceived as confusing. Despite assurances that there is no calorie counting or banned foods, the plan does impose portion control through the size of servings and caloric restriction.

treats

PICK FROM:
- 1 biscuit pack (100 calories)
- 7 chocolate-covered almonds
- 30g fudge
- 20 corn candy
- 55g angel cake
- 2 pieces of Kit Kat chocolate
- 20 peanuts
- string cheese

Is it for you?

The structured eating plan of the 3-Hour Diet will attract people who like to snack and are into fitness. Those with a medical condition for which amounts of food, frequency of eating, or taking time-controlled medications are key considerations should consult a doctor first.

Availability

Most foods in this diet can be bought in any general food shop or supermarket.

Lifestyle changes

Alongside regular exercise, the plan encourages visualization techniques, strategies for "loser zones" (time wasters), "targets" (reasons for weight loss), "hungry heart" (emotional eating), "support pillars" (positive past accomplishments), People Solution™ (support network) and a "positive (self) name tag".

free foods

Any foods less than 20 calories per serving.
- pickles
- lime juice
- jicama
- green onions
- lettuce
- radishes
- cucumber
- courgettes

snacks about 100 calories.

	wednesday	thursday	friday
	egg muffin, 1 glass orange juice	grilled cheese sandwich, apple, ½ glass pineapple juice	ham omelette, ½ bagel, 2 figs, 240ml cranberry juice cocktail
	chicken fajita pitta, cucumber slices, fat-free ranch dressing, 1% milk	pizza (400 calories, frozen), broccoli and sprout salad, 1 tsp olive oil	cheese cannelloni (400 calories, entrée), green salad, 1 tsp flaxseed oil
	ham and bean soup, beetroot, onion roll	baked trout, redskin potatoes with vegetables, 2 tbsp flaxseed	turkey chilli, mixed carrots and parsnips, green salad, 1 tsp flaxseed oil
	1 low-fat string cheese	apple sauce	small brownie
	55g angel cake, green tea	low-fat muesli bar	12 almonds, green tea
	6 cashews, cucumber sticks	5 mini rice cakes 2 tsp low-sugar jam	5 small cheddar crisps

Resources

www.jorgecruise.com

www.everydiet.org/3_hour_diet.htm

Cruise, J. *The 3-Hour Diet* (2006, HarperCollins)

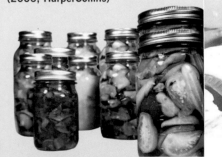

LONG-TERM PLAN

FLEXIBILITY

FAMILY FRIENDLY

COST

STRENGTH OF SCIENCE

NEW BEVERLY HILLS DIET

This 35-day programme emphasizes strict food combinations at specific times of the day.

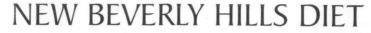

Diet history
Created by Judy Mazel and first published in 1981, the original Beverly Hills Diet was revised in the 1990s as the New Beverly Hills Diet. Although well known for a time, the American Dietetic Association and the American Medical Association spoke out against its principles. The book, however, is still in print and available from online bookstores and public libraries.

How does it work?
The plan is based on a 35-day programme during which only fruit may be consumed for breakfast. The quantity of fruit allowed is unlimited but only one type of fruit can be eaten at a time, followed by a second type one hour later. The person dieting must then wait a further two to three hours before eating a food from any other food group, and this cannot be followed by more fruit. If the next kind of food to be eaten is a carbohydrate, only carbohydrates can be eaten after that albeit in any amount.

Grains, vegetables and salads are classified as carbohydrates. Wine, brandy, champagne and cognac are considered fruits, while beer and

weigh this up...
• The five-week daily diary included in the book will be helpful for anyone who wants to stick closely to the diet.

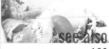

see also
suzanne somers 120

sample menu

There is an abundance of fruit allowed, but with

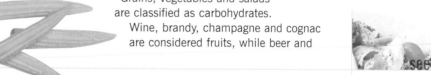

	saturday	sunday	monday	tuesday
8am	watermelon	230g dried apricots	strawberries	pineapple
10am (or 2 hours later)	2 bananas	kiwi	strawberries	papaya
12–1pm (or 2–3 hours later)	corn-on-the-cob, lettuce salad with chickpeas, peppers and olive oil	baked potato with sour cream and green onions, relish tray with radishes, carrots and broccoli	avocado, tomato and onion sandwich on wholewheat bread, cooked cabbage	asparagus, celery and courgette stir-fry, rice
after 3–4pm (rest of the day)	steak, eggs	deli meat platter with pastrami, ham and a variety of cheeses	steamed oysters, lamb chops, ice cream	combination plate of chicken salad, tuna salad and egg salad

spirits are also labelled as carbohydrates. Once protein is introduced, 80 per cent of food intake must be protein. Carbohydrates and proteins can never be combined.

The plan's rationale is that it is possible to lose between 4.5–7kg (10–15lb) during the duration of the programme. By not combining certain kinds of foods together, the enzymes in one particular type of food (when not eaten in combination with other types of food) cause it to be inefficiently digested. The scientific evidence, however, does not support this assertion. Weight loss may be rapid but dieters probably lose the pounds from the reduced food intake, corresponding calorie drop and loss of water.

Pros and cons

The diet plan promotes an abundant consumption of fruit (which provides water), fibre and vital nutrients such as vitamins A and C. Nevertheless, consuming fruit in such quantities can lead to diarrhoea, which has the potential to cause dehydration. The Beverly Hills Diet does have the potential for deficiencies in protein, calcium, iron and B group vitamins. Some dieters may feel the programme lacks sufficient guidance as there is no portion control and any scientific evidence in support of the regime is lacking.

Is it for you?

People with a lot of time to plan meals will enjoy going on the Beverly Hills Diet the most. A solid understanding of food-combining principles is necessary and anyone who does not learn the diet's principles by heart will struggle. Individuals with gastrointestinal conditions for which a low-fibre or low-residue diet is recommended should avoid it.

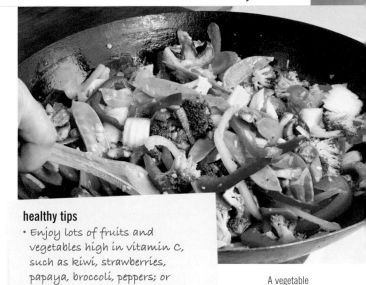

healthy tips
- Enjoy lots of fruits and vegetables high in vitamin C, such as kiwi, strawberries, papaya, broccoli, peppers; or fruits and vegetables rich in vitamin A, such as cantaloupe, dried apricots, mango, sweet potato and carrots.

A vegetable stir-fry with rice is considered a carbohydrate meal.

Availability

Most foods in this diet are widely available but certain kinds of fruit and the vast quantities required for a constant supply may prove expensive for some.

Lifestyle changes

The programme recommends five minutes of daily exercise.

restrictions on combinations and times.

wednesday	thursday	friday
grapes	170g prunes	cherries
grapes	blueberries	mango
wholewheat bagels with tomato, shallots, green and red pepper rings and olive oil	lettuce, tomato and onion sandwich on rye bread, French fries	chipotle salsa, taco chips, beer
hamburger, eggs	230g raw brazil nuts, yogurt	baked salmon, cheesecake

Note: Unless specified, amounts are as desired.

Resources

www.skinnyondiets.com

Mazel, J., Wyatt, M.
The New Beverly Hills Diet
(1996, Health Communications)

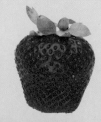

LONG-TERM PLAN

FLEXIBILITY

FAMILY FRIENDLY

COST

STRENGTH OF SCIENCE

FIT FOR LIFE

This disciplined timing and food combination plan claims to improve digestion and increase metabolism to promote weight loss.

Diet history
Published in 1985, the highly publicized plan by Harvey and Marilyn Diamond was followed up by *Fit for Life II: Living Health* (1987).

How does it work?
The central premise of Fit for Life is that nutrition depends more on when and what you eat rather than how much you eat. The consumption of specific food combinations in the course of the day is claimed to enhance nutrient absorption by the gastrointestinal tract and result in a higher rate of metabolism.

The plan dictates that a high percentage of calories should come from fruit and vegetables with dairy, grains, meat products and foods containing refined sugar severely restricted. Although the programme does not place major emphasis on the total amount of calories consumed, it does stress the importance of not overeating and asserts that certain foods eaten in inappropriate combinations can trigger specific physiological reactions that interfere with the absorption of

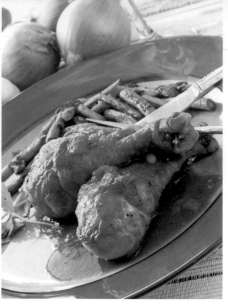

Lean meat or poultry and vegetables for dinner make meal planning simple.

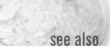

see also
suzanne somers 120

sample menu
The rigorous restrictions and food combinations

	saturday	sunday	monday	tuesday
morning	freshly squeezed juice, fresh fruit or fruit salad	strawberry-kiwi salad with orange and banana	freshly squeezed juice, fresh fruit or fruit salad	freshly squeezed juice, fresh fruit or fruit salad
lunch	cauliflower spread with celery, bean sprouts and carrots on 1 slice wholegrain bread	grilled cucumber and lettuce wrapped in corn tortilla	salad of lettuce, spinach, cucumber, tomato, bean sprouts, olives and green beans	vegetable fruit platter with tomato, cucumber and avocado
supper	carrot hash browns, teriyaki broccoli, tangy green coleslaw	fresh vegetable juice, shepherd's pie with vegetables, carrots with basil, carrot salad with asparagus	fresh vegetable juice, cauliflower soup, roast chicken, string beans with garlic, green salad	fresh vegetable juice, papaya, Mediterranean-style rice salad with courgette, lettuce, rocket, bean sprouts and green olives
snack 1	fresh fruit or carrot juice	fresh fruit or carrot juice	fresh fruit or carrot juice	fresh fruit or carrot juice
snack 2	fruit snack 3 hours after dinner	fruit snack 3 hours after dinner	fruit snack 3 hours after dinner	fruit snack 3 hours after dinner

nutrients and the release of toxins. The release of toxins is believed to produce weight gain as the enzymes required to digest the different types of food counteract one another.

Breakfast consists solely of fruit or fruit juice. Lunchtime includes fruit, salads or vegetables and allows occasional grains such as an "energy salad" or a "properly combined sandwich". Dinner is a combination of fruit, vegetables and lean meats.

It is these rigorous restrictions which cause the reduction in calories and weight.

Pros and cons

High in fruit and vegetables, the Fit for Life Diet restricts the consumption of fats from animal sources but lets you enjoy any amount of fresh fruit, fruit juice, vegetables and lean meats. Unfortunately, the programme is nutritionally flawed as it fails to provide the dieter with an adequate range of nutrients, including protein, zinc, vitamin D and vitamin B12. So far, all of its claims, including the underlying theory (that the enzyme activity from specific food groups being metabolized triggers a digestive conflict that can cause weight gain), have yet to be supported by scientific evidence.

Is it for you?

The Fit for Life Plan is likely to attract those who enjoy having a lot of fruit and vegetables and are happy to follow a rigid eating plan. The prospect of weight loss due

weigh this up...
• Fit for Life is a weight-loss plan that does not involve any counting of calories, but emphasizes avoiding overeating.

to caloric restrictions may be appealing, but without lifestyle changes and a more balanced meal plan to match, this can only be a short-term fix. Anyone with a medical condition should be aware of the diet's nutritional deficiencies and healthy individuals should follow it for a short period of time only.

Availability

All the foods in this diet can be readily bought from any general food store or supermarket.

Lifestyle changes

The plan emphasizes the importance of not overeating and suggests that a high water content cleanses the body, unclogs the intestines and increases nutrient absorption to reduce cravings.

forbidden foods

- refined sugars
- dairy products
- most meat products
- vinegar in salad dressings
- white (non-wholegrain) breads

require advanced planning.

wednesday	thursday	friday
freshly squeezed juice, fresh fruit or fruit salad	freshly squeezed juice, fresh fruit or fruit salad	freshly squeezed juice, fresh fruit or fruit salad
fresh fruit or carrot juice (optional), raw vegetables with butternut squash dip	fresh fruit or carrot juice (optional), plain nuts, cucumber	vegetable-fruit platter with tomato, cucumber, and avocado
corn chowder, New York Goodwich of steamed vegetables and barbecue onions in a tortilla	fresh vegetable juice, vegetable stew, curried cabbage, Caesar salad	cantaloupe, curried chicken salad
fresh fruit or carrot juice	fresh fruit or carrot juice	fresh fruit or carrot juice
fruit snack 3 hours after dinner	fruit snack 3 hours after dinner	fruit snack 3 hours after dinner

Resources

www.fitforlife.com

Diamond, H., Diamond, M. *Fit for Life* (1985, Warner Books)

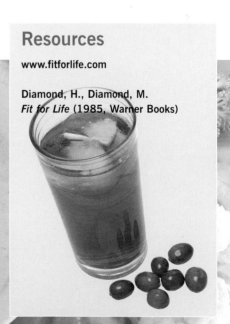

Note: All recipes in the plan are available in *Fit for Life*.

LONG-TERM PLAN
● ● ●

FLEXIBILITY
● ● ●

FAMILY FRIENDLY
●

COST
●

STRENGTH OF SCIENCE
● ●

GRAZING DIET

This guide to healthy snacking requires careful planning to ensure all daily nutrient requirements are met in the course of the six or seven small meals allowed.

Diet history
Once popular back in the nineties, the Grazing Diet has since lost widespread appeal.

How does it work?
The rationale is that small amounts of food eaten on a regular basis curb hunger and food cravings by stabilizing blood sugar and insulin levels and averting fluctuations. There is no need for "treats" as all foods are allowed and the body burns calories during digestion so several small meals help to keep an active metabolic rate. Grazing is not about having milk and biscuits but about finding non-fattening and creative ways to enrich your diet with protein, complex carbohydrates, vitamins and minerals.

Pros and cons
Grazing or healthy snacking differs from the usual eating habits of the Western world but is fast becoming the American way of eating.

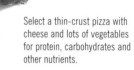

Select a thin-crust pizza with cheese and lots of vegetables for protein, carbohydrates and other nutrients.

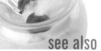

see also
3-hour 110

sample menu
Keys to success are careful planning and

	saturday	sunday	monday	tuesday
morning	2 buckwheat pancakes, strawberry sauce, ⅛ honeydew melon	burrito on flour tortilla, black beans and salsa, 110ml skimmed milk, ½ grapefruit	100g porridge, raisins, 120ml low-fat milk, 120ml orange juice	50g bran flakes, 120ml low-fat milk, 1 banana, 120ml prune juice
snack 1	fat-free fruit yogurt, 2 wholewheat breadsticks	orange, fat-free yogurt, 4 wholewheat crackers,	orange, 100g fat-free yogurt, 2 crackers	1 peanut butter-filled celery stick, strawberries
lunch	1 slice pizza, Caesar salad, low-fat dressing, water	240ml split pea and mushroom soup, wholewheat toast, water	½ turkey sandwich on rye bread, lettuce, low-fat mayo, water	½ tuna fish sandwich on wholewheat bread, lettuce, tomato, water
snack 2	2 tbsp hummus, wholewheat bread, fruit cocktail	½ peanut butter sandwich, skimmed milk	1 apple, 80g mixed almonds, walnuts and pistachios	pear, plain fat-free yogurt, 4 crackers, skimmed milk
supper	vegetable stir-fry with tofu, bok choy and pepper, 200g brown rice, 1 apple, water	Spanish rice with seafood, grilled aubergine and courgette, green salad, plums and peaches	spinach lasagne, green salad, wholewheat bread, margarine, cantaloupe, water	½ chicken breast, sweet potatoes, peas and onions, 100g brown rice, spinach, bean salad
snack 3	40g sunflower seeds, banana, skimmed milk	mixed dried fruit and nuts, fat-free yogurt	½ egg salad sandwich, fat-free fruit yogurt	dried prunes, apricots and raisins, fat-free yogurt

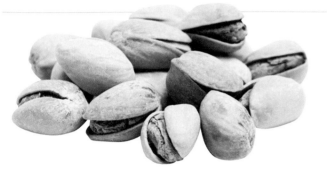

It helps fill in those necessary calories and nutrients you might otherwise miss due to incomplete or skipped meals. Eating small, frequent meals gives the individual a sense of satiety by keeping the physiological balance between blood sugar and insulin levels. When planned correctly, grazing prevents compulsive overeating and excessive calorie consumption.

Meeting the necessary daily requirements, however, requires careful planning. Potential grazers should work with a dietician to set up a daily menu that is within their calorie goals. Grazing can disrupt a family's routine, as the traditional pattern of three meals and a snack may be more convenient. A grazing eating pattern may also interfere with work because it is time-consuming to plan and must be carefully done or it could lead to overeating and excessive caloric intake. Erratic snacking should not be confused with a carefully monitored grazing plan, which requires portion control.

Is it for you?
Grazing is most likely to appeal to a single person with the time and knowledge necessary to plan and execute the diet with success. This method of dieting is not harmful but does require planning. It is always best to consult a dietician before embarking on this diet. How you graze and what you choose to snack on will depend on your age and lifestyle. Variations of the plan are also advocated for treating medical conditions which require frequent eating or for post-gastric surgery (gastric bypass, reduction and gastrectomy).

Availability
All the foods in this diet are widely available and can be readily purchased from a general food store or supermarket.

Lifestyle changes
Exercise and a change in eating patterns is essential.

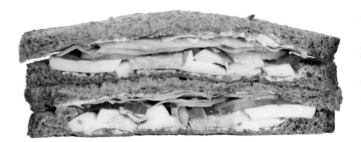

portion control.

wednesday	thursday	friday	Resources
½ muffin, butter, jam, ½ grapefruit, 1 hard-boiled egg	25g cold cereal, skimmed milk, banana, wholewheat toast	2 slices French toast, apple sauce, skimmed milk, ½ grapefruit	**diet.ivillage.com/issues/isnacks/0,,1khs,00.html**
mixed nuts, banana, fat-free yogurt	orange, 110g cottage cheese, 2 crackers	grapes, tomatoes, carrot, 4 wholewheat crackers	**Mitchell, S. and Christie, C.** *I'd Kill For a Cookie* (1998, Plume)
240ml vegetable and bean soup, bread sticks, orange, water	½ toasted cheese sandwich, carrot, tomatoes, water	240ml lentil soup, wholewheat toast, spring vegetable salad, apple	
fat-free fruit yogurt, carrot and celery sticks	fruit salad, crackers	fat-free yogurt, 60g soya nuts, 1 cucumber	
rigatoni with meat sauce, spinach and nut salad, light vinaigrette dressing, tangerine, water	80g grilled steak, steamed carrots, green beans, baked potato, fat-free plain yogurt	pizza with thick-cut bacon, onion and mushrooms, green salad, 100g blueberries	
25g cereal, skimmed milk, blackberries	breadsticks, 15g cheese, cantaloupe	skimmed milk, wholewheat crackers	

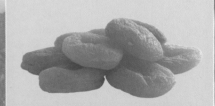

LONG-TERM PLAN
●

FLEXIBILITY
●

FAMILY FRIENDLY
●

COST
●

STRENGTH OF SCIENCE
●

HAY DIET

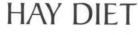

This eating guide promotes weight loss by avoiding food combinations like starches with proteins and acid fruits at the same meal.

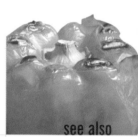

Diet history
Formerly the Food Combining Diet, the Hay Diet was inspired by the dietary principles of Dr William Howard Hay which were published in the 1935 edition of *Health via Food*.

How does it work?
This food-combining programme suggests that a wide range of health problems result from the body's accumulation of toxins and acid waste products when combining starches and proteins at the same meal, eating too many acid-forming proteins, starches, processed foods and too few alkaline-forming vegetables and fruit. Everything that we eat has either an acid-forming or alkaline-forming effect so food combining maintains the right digestive equilibrium. According to the Hay Diet, the key to good health is to reduce the amount of acidity-forming foods and increase the presence of beneficial, alkaline-forming foods.

The following eating pattern should be followed to maintain the body's balance: one completely alkaline-forming meal (fruit and vegetables only), one starch meal and one protein meal. Vegetables,

see also
fit for life 114
suzanne somers 120

sample menu
For the fasting regime from Friday evening to

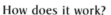

	saturday	sunday	monday	tuesday
morning	clementines (fasting detox)	cheese omelette	wholewheat muffins with honey	porridge
lunch	honeydew (fasting detox)	Chinese vegetable stir-fry	baked chicken breast with roasted vegetables	tropical fruit salad
supper	baked potato with sautéed mushrooms	wholewheat pasta with tomatoes and artichoke hearts	spinach salad with grapes and tomatoes	flounder with broccoli and cauliflower
snack 1	cherries	apple juice	fruit juice	tomato salad
snack 2	watermelon	almonds	carrot sticks	peach

weigh this up...

- In the Hay Diet, proteins include all kinds of meats and cheeses, yogurt, milk, eggs, fish, poultry and soya products. Starches include grains, such as rice, pasta, breads, crackers, biscuits and all types of sugars and white flour with the exception of soya flour, which is considered a protein.

salads and fruits are alkaline and neutral so can be mixed with all of the food groups and eaten alongside any meal as the main part of the diet. Eat proteins, starches and fats in small quantities and only wholegrain and unprocessed starches excluding refined, processed foods. Allow an interval of at least four to four and a half hours between meals of different types for optimal digestion.

This dietary system also includes a weekly fast or detox regime which consists of fresh salads and fruit (from Friday evening to Saturday afternoon) to flush out the accumulated toxins and aid digestion.

In spite of its logical rationale, there is little hard scientific evidence to support the Hay Diet. According to science, the human body is resilient and able to digest foods in any combination, at any time. Weight loss is achieved on this plan because of the caloric restrictions imposed on eating certain food groups together, not from the specific combinations themselves.

Pros and cons

Food combining principles may be attractive to dieters who desire weight loss without calorie counting. The Hay Diet promotes eating a lot of fruit and vegetables, which can only be beneficial for anyone. It can, however, be extremely restrictive and confusing with the time allowed between fruit, proteins and starches. The weekly fresh fruit and vegetable detox is very limiting.

Is it for you?

This diet will appeal to individuals who enjoy plant-based foods or to individuals who prefer to follow limited food lists. Those with diabetes or any other medical condition should consult a doctor about the restriction on calories and food groups.

Availability

All of the foods in this diet can be bought in any general food shop or supermarket.

Lifestyle changes

Unhealthy activities such as smoking and overworking plus harmful mental states such as stress and negative thoughts are all acid forming.

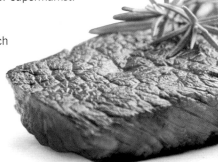

Saturday, eat only fresh salads and fruits.

wednesday	thursday	friday	Resources
crunchy homemade muesli	grapefruit	cantaloupe	www.thedietchannel.com/Food-combining.htm
roasted peppers with sautéed Swiss chard	vegetable soup with wholewheat baguette	tuna salad on salad greens	Marsden, K. *The Food Combining Diet: Lose Weight the Hay Way* (1993, Thorsons)
grilled sirloin with asparagus	roasted turkey breast with green salad	raw vegetables (fasting detox)	
strawberries	kiwi fruit	blueberries	
carrot juice	guacamole with crudités	tomato juice	

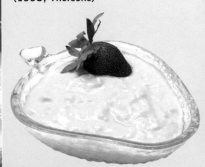

SUZANNE SOMERS DIET

Based on the principle that controlling the amount of insulin released after a meal is necessary to achieving weight loss, this food-focused plan exercises dietary control through specific meal combinations.

LONG-TERM PLAN

FLEXIBILITY

FAMILY FRIENDLY

COST ●

STRENGTH OF SCIENCE

Diet history

First published by US actress Suzanne Somers but originally based on the Schwarzbein Principle – that degenerative diseases of ageing are the result of imbalance and poor eating and lifestyle habits – this diet is also labelled Somerizing or Somersizing. Ms Somers has written further books related to the diet.

How does it work?

According to this diet, fat does not make you fat, sugar is more fattening than fat, and carbohydrates are not essential. Weight gain is caused by hormonal imbalances and successful weight loss depends on keeping the release of insulin stable following digestion.

This is achieved by eating certain foods in specific combinations, cutting down on carbs, and eliminating sugars, starchy foods, white flour, caffeine and "funky foods". The person dieting should never skip meals and is allowed fruit, proteins, carbohydrates and fats with certain vegetables, followed by a three-hour interval between any protein, fat or carbohydrate meal. After eating fruit, the dieter should wait 20 minutes before consuming any other foods. Refined carbohydrates are totally excluded, although some fibre-rich complex carbohydrates are featured at key stages.

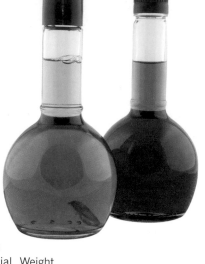

Spinach and peppers (right) are rich in phytochemicals and low in calories.

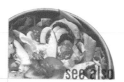

see also
3-hour 110
fit for life 114
hay 118

sample menu

There is a three-hour interval between any

	saturday	sunday	monday	tuesday
morning	buckwheat pancakes	asparagus frittata	½ cantaloupe, omelette, bacon, courgette	wholegrain toast, low-fat cottage cheese
lunch	picadillo, roasted aubergine and peppers, shiitake mushroom soup	grilled scallops, steamed green beans and celery root	roasted pork loin, chanterelles with parmesan and olive oil, spinach salad	lemon pepper chicken strips, sautéed summer squash, green salad
supper	grilled steak, grilled aubergine, courgette and squash side salad	chicken kebabs, grilled peppers, Greek salad with feta cheese	tuna with greens, bamboo shoots, hearts of palm, ginger, sesame oil, wine vinegar	pitta and hummus, cucumber and parsley salad, roasted aubergine
snack 1	pineapple and apricot salad	lychee and loquat salad	pear and apple salad	grapefruit and orange salad
snack 2	fruit smoothie	salsa, jicama slices	veggie dip, carrot sticks	fruit smoothie

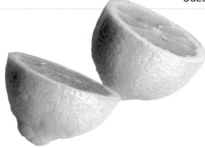

There are two levels to this eating guide. Level One is the most restrictive and designed to initiate weight loss. Level Two is the maintenance phase and introduces some protein, fat and carbohydrate combinations. Portion control is key, so it stands to reason that the resulting weight loss is probably due to the total caloric intake of structured meals instead of the food combinations.

Pros and cons

The plan promotes structured meals, moderate portion sizes and the consumption of fruit and vegetables. Its creative menu provides not just healthy but also tasty options and the large quantity of fruit and vegetables supply the dieter with the necessary bulk and fluid.

However, the rationale for the diet's effectiveness is not substantiated by any of the scientific data and some of its statements are incorrect. For example, sugar (which provides four calories per gram or about 20 calories for a level teaspoon) is not more fattening than fat (which provides nine calories per gram or about 45 calories per level teaspoon). In general, food can be consumed in various combinations without any detrimental effects.

Is it for you?

This celebrity diet will attract individuals who look up to famous role models, like to snack on fruit, and/or are able to carefully plan a menu since the restrictions related to the food combinations can be time consuming. Those with medical conditions (such as diabetes) should avoid this diet.

Availability

Most foods in this diet can be purchased from general food shops or supermarkets.

Lifestyle changes

Regular exercise is recommended.

forbidden foods

- most sugars
- white flour
- white rice
- bananas
- corn
- carrots
- beetroot
- pumpkin
- potatoes, yams and sweet potatoes
- parsnips
- caffeine
- alcohol

free foods

- soy sauce
- vinegar
- mustard
- herbs
- lemons
- limes

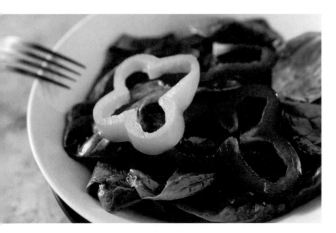

carbohydrate, protein or fat meal.

wednesday	thursday	friday
scrambled egg with prawns and mushroom	smoothie, (wait 20 minutes), wholewheat toast	boiled egg, sausage, grilled tomato
grilled salmon, steamed broccoli, lettuce and goat's cheese salad	grilled steak, salsa, garden greens, tomatoes	baked cod, cauliflower soup, spinach salad with olive oil and vinegar
wholewheat pasta with tomato sauce and cheese	brown rice and black beans, tossed green salad, green beans	vegetable wholewheat lasagne, romano cheese, cobb salad
mixed berry salad	mango, papaya slices	watermelon
salsa, celery sticks	apple and grape salad	veggie dip, pepper strips

Resources

www.suzannesomers.com

Somers, S. *Suzanne Somers' Fast and Easy* (2002, Crown Publications)

Somers, S. *Get Skinny on Fabulous Food* (1999, Crown Publications)

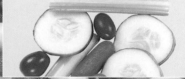

LONG-TERM PLAN

FLEXIBILITY

FAMILY FRIENDLY

COST

STRENGTH OF SCIENCE

THE ULTRASIMPLE DIET

This weight-loss diet is based on the premise that obesity is due to inflammation and toxicity of the body.

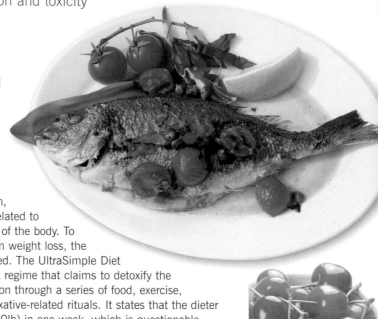

Diet history
This is a more recent and shorter variation of the author's original and popular diet, the *UltraMetabolism Diet* (Mark Hyman, 2006).

How does it work?
According to this diet plan, obesity and disease are related to toxicity and inflammation of the body. To achieve effective long-term weight loss, the body needs to be detoxified. The UltraSimple Diet is a quick-start, one-week regime that claims to detoxify the body and cool inflammation through a series of food, exercise, supplement intake and laxative-related rituals. It states that the dieter could safely lose 4½kg (10lb) in one week, which is questionable.

see also
suzanne somers 120
perricone 168

sample menu
This plan emphasizes a one-week detox

	saturday	sunday	monday	tuesday
snack 1	2 tsp organic extra virgin olive oil and ½ organic lemon drink	2 tsp organic extra virgin olive oil and ½ organic lemon drink	2 tsp organic extra virgin olive oil and ½ organic lemon drink	2 tsp organic extra virgin olive oil and ½ organic lemon drink
morning	lemon juice and hot water, 240ml green tea, UltraShake	lemon juice and hot water, 240ml green tea, UltraShake	lemon juice and hot water, 240ml green tea, UltraShake	lemon juice and hot water, 240ml green tea, UltraShake
snack 2	240ml UltraBroth, UltraShake without flaxseeds (optional)	240ml UltraBroth, UltraShake without flaxseeds (optional)	240ml UltraBroth, UltraShake without flaxseeds (optional)	240ml UltraBroth, UltraShake without flaxseeds (optional)
lunch	steamed vegetables, 100g brown rice, UltraShake (optional)	steamed vegetables, 100g brown rice, 50g fruit or berries, UltraShake (optional)	steamed vegetables, 100g brown rice, 50g fruit or berries, UltraShake (optional)	steamed vegetables, 100g brown rice, UltraShake (optional)
snack 3	240ml UltraBroth, UltraShake (optional)	240ml UltraBroth, UltraShake (optional)	240ml UltraBroth	240ml UltraBroth, UltraShake (optional)
dinner	400g lightly sautéed vegetables, 100g brown rice, 110–170g fish, 240ml UltraBroth	400g sautéed vegetables, 100g brown rice, 110–170g chicken breast, 240ml UltraBroth	400g lightly sautéed vegetables, 100g brown rice, 110–170g fish, 240ml UltraBroth	400g sautéed vegetables, 100g brown rice, 110–170g chicken breast, 240ml UltraBroth

The book contains detailed information about what to do from day one through to day seven, and how to move out of the diet. Basically, it is a low-calorie plan that includes recipes for an UltraBroth and UltraShake, along with very structured exercise and relaxation activities, instructions for taking specific supplements and laxatives, and for using a sauna or steam room and taking relaxing baths. The person must plan an approximate two-hour ritual of "detoxification", yoga, special midmorning, lunch, afternoon and dinner foods and supplements, then specified exercise and bedtime detoxification, more exercise and journaling rituals. The weight loss is likely due to the diet's low calorie level, water loss and the use of laxatives.

Pros and cons

This highly regimented plan will appeal to persons who like a lot of structure and guidance. There is a shopping list included, which will facilitate getting the items needed for this diet. The dieter must be willing to take the special "detox" herbs and other supplements, and follow the rituals for taking laxatives.

Is it for you?

This diet is likely to appeal to persons who like detoxification rituals and do not mind the frequent use of laxatives. All persons with any health condition should consult a doctor before trying this diet, especially if on medications for which some supplements or other items on this diet might be harmful.

Availability

Some of the foods can be bought in any general food store, but the dieter may need to go to a pharmacy for some items, such as the probiotic capsules, filtered waters and magnesium citrate, and to a special shop for some organic products and the detox supportive herbs.

Lifestyle changes

The plan is restrictive, and lifestyle undergoes a considerable one-week change, so the dieter must have a flexible week to follow the diet.

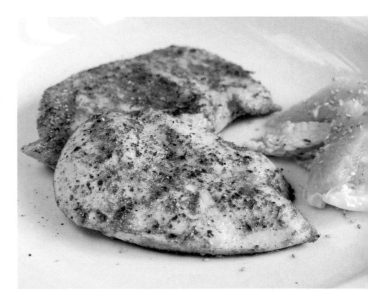

regime that includes UltraBroths.

wednesday	thursday	friday
2 tsp organic extra virgin olive oil and ½ organic lemon drink	2 tsp organic extra virgin olive oil and ½ organic lemon drink	2 tsp organic extra virgin olive oil and ½ organic lemon drink
lemon juice and hot water, 240ml green tea, UltraShake	lemon juice and hot water, 240ml green tea, UltraShake	lemon juice and hot water, 240ml green tea, UltraShake
240ml UltraBroth, UltraShake without flaxseeds (optional)	240ml UltraBroth, UltraShake without flaxseeds (optional)	240ml UltraBroth, UltraShake without flaxseeds (optional)
steamed vegetables, 100g brown rice, UltraShake (optional)	steamed vegetables, 100g brown rice, UltraShake (optional)	steamed vegetables, 100g brown rice, UltraShake (optional)
240ml UltraBroth, UltraShake (optional)	240ml UltraBroth, UltraShake (optional)	240ml UltraBroth, UltraShake (optional)
400g lightly sautéed vegetables, 100g brown rice, 110–170g fish, 240ml UltraBroth	400g lightly sautéed vegetables, 100g brown rice, 110–170g legumes, 240ml UltraBroth	400g lightly sautéed vegetables, 100g brown rice, 110–170g tofu, 240ml UltraBroth

Resources

http://ultrametabolism.com

Hyman, M. *The UltraSimple Diet* (2007, Pocket Books, Simon & Schuster)

Hyman, M. *UltraMetabolism* (2006, Simon & Schuster)

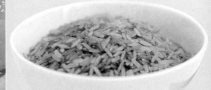

Note: The supplements or laxatives indicated as part of some mealtimes are not included in this plan, but details are available in *The UltraSimple Diet.*

LONG-TERM PLAN
●●

FLEXIBILITY
●

FAMILY FRIENDLY
●

COST
●

STRENGTH OF SCIENCE
●

EAT RIGHT FOR YOUR TYPE

The book is organized into four diets, designed for the four blood types, claiming to provide the diet solution to staying healthy, living longer and achieving ideal weight.

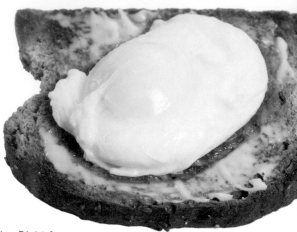

Diet history
Eat Right for Your Type was developed by naturopath Peter D'Adamo, ND, who is the founder and editor emeritus of *The Journal of Naturopathic Medicine*, and author of *Live Right for Your Type* and *Cook Right for Your Type*. Introduced in 1996, the book and its sequels were all on the *New York Times* bestseller list.

Ezekiel bread with poached egg (for type AB).

How does it work?
There are four diets based on the blood types O, A, B and AB. People with type O are described as hunters, who need a diet with lean high protein, chemical-free meat, poultry and fish, with limited grains, beans and legumes. Those with type A blood, the cultivators, need to eat predominantly vegetarian, with fish, and the emphasis on vegetables, tofu, grains, beans, legumes and fruit. Type B, the

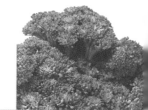

sample menu
A menu is provided for each blood-type diet.

	type A	type AB	type B	type O
morning	water with lemon, cornflakes with soya milk and blueberries, grapefruit juice, coffee or herbal tea	water with lemon, 225ml diluted grapefruit juice, 1 slice Ezekiel bread, 1 poached egg	rice bran cereal with banana and skimmed milk	puffed rice with soya milk, 1 poached egg, 225ml pineapple juice, green or herbal tea
lunch	Greek salad, apple, 1 slice wheat bread, herbal tea	110g turkey breast, 1 slice rye bread, Caesar salad, 2 plums, herbal tea	spinach salad, 110g water-packed tuna, 2 rice cakes, herbal tea	110g grilled minced beef patty, 2 slices Essene bread, salad with olive oil and lemon juice, water or herbal tea
supper	tofu stir-fry with green beans, leeks, mange-tout, alfalfa sprouts, coffee or herbal tea	tofu omelette, stir-fried vegetables, mixed fruit salad, decaf coffee	grilled fish, steamed vegetables, sweet potato, fresh fruit, herbal tea or coffee	grilled minced lamb patty, chicory salad, herbal tea
snack	2 rice cakes with honey, 2 plums, green tea or water	110ml low-fat yogurt with fruit	low-fat yogurt with raisins	mixed fruit, herbal tea

nomads, should eat meat (no chicken), dairy, grains, beans, legumes, vegetables and fruit. Type AB, the enigma, can eat a mixed diet in moderation, including meat, seafood, dairy, tofu, beans, legumes, grains, vegetables and fruit.

The author describes the presence of protein "lectins" in specific foods, which are incompatible with a particular blood type antigens, so they target an organ or bodily system (kidneys, liver, brain and so on) and begin to "agglutinate" blood cells in that area. Each blood type has its own list of foods that should be avoided based on this theory, with a long list of "forbidden" foods in each category, including meats and poultry, seafood, dairy, eggs, oils and fats, nuts and seeds, beans, legumes, cereals, breads, muffins, grains, pasta, vegetables, fruit, juices, fluids, spices, condiments, herbal teas and other beverages.

Pros and cons
All the diets consist of whole, unprocessed foods and all recommend the consumption of vegetables, which provide fibre, many health-promoting nutrients and phytochemicals.

However, there is no scientific validity to the idea that diet should be defined by blood type. By limiting particular foods (and sometimes food groups), those who follow the diet can successfully lose weight, but they are eliminating specific foods and groups based on a premise without adequate scientific evidence.

healthy tips
- What are lectins?
Lectins are complex molecules that have both protein and sugars that are able to bind to the outside of a cell and cause biochemical changes in it. Lectins are made by both animals and plants. However, the role of lectins, and claims made regarding its relation to blood typing, diet and disease prevention, are not established by current scientific data.

forbidden foods
Each blood type has its own list of foods that should be avoided.

Is it for you?
The type O diet places high emphasis on meat, while limiting grains, beans and legumes. This could be unhealthy for those with a family history of heart disease, hypertension and diabetes, as it is counter to current recommendations for prevention and treatment of these diseases.

Availability
Depending on blood type, different foods are recommended; however, most are generally available.

Lifestyle changes
Physical activity, stress management and reducing health risks in the environment are integrated in the plan.

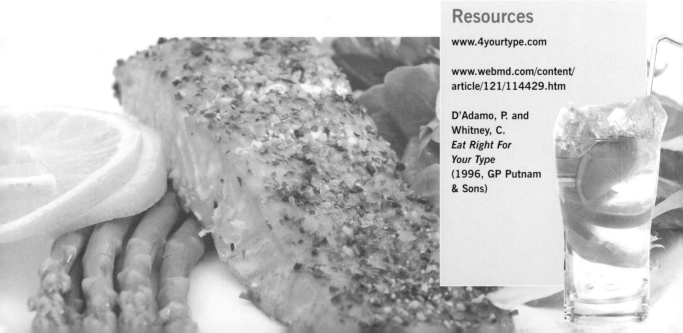

Resources
www.4yourtype.com

www.webmd.com/content/ article/121/114429.htm

D'Adamo, P. and Whitney, C. *Eat Right For Your Type* (1996, GP Putnam & Sons)

LONG-TERM PLAN

FLEXIBILITY

FAMILY FRIENDLY

COST
●

STRENGTH OF SCIENCE

FASTING DIET

The oldest and most radical of diets, fasting is the practice of refraining from eating food alongside the sole consumption of water or juice.

Diet history

The origins of fasting as a weight-loss method are lost in the mists of time, but it has probably been practised since the dawn of civilization for a number of non-dietary reasons. These probably included food scarcity, religious ritual, or simply as a method of cleansing the body physically and spiritually, with weight loss as a side effect.

The practice of fasting followed by a period of extreme overeating is culturally acceptable in certain societies where large groups of people fast for a specific reason and often end it by participating in festivities or rituals that involve an excessive consumption of food.

How does it work?

The rationale behind a fast is that the total avoidance of food provides a quick weight-loss method. In some cultures, this practice serves as a form of penitence for overindulgence and has religious overtones.

Without food, blood sugar levels go down as no essential fuel in the form of energy is entering the body. This dip is registered and a neurochemical message is sent to the brain promoting hunger pangs to kick in. During a fast, feelings of hunger come and go as the body is reminding you that you will need to eat at some point. During the first few hours of the fast, the body will obtain energy or glucose either from the glycogen stored in the muscles (only for use by the muscles) or the liver (for use by the rest of the body). This energy reserve lasts

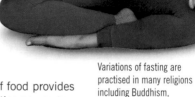

Variations of fasting are practised in many religions including Buddhism, Hinduism, Islam, Bahai and Christianity.

see also
juicing 90

sample menu

This menu progresses to a fasting diet, which

	saturday	sunday	monday	tuesday
morning	porridge with raisins and margarine, fat-free milk, grape juice	wholewheat muffin, jam, orange segments, egg, tea	wholewheat muffin, jam, orange segments, egg, tea	French toast with maple syrup, ½ grapefruit, fat-free milk
lunch	taco salad with minced turkey, beans and low-fat cheese	tuna sandwich on rye bread with lettuce and tomato, pear, fat-free milk	white bean soup, breadsticks, carrot sticks, fat-free milk	rigatoni with tomato sauce, spinach salad, fat-free milk
supper	beet lasagne, wholewheat dinner roll, fat-free milk	roasted chicken breast baked sweet potatoes, peas, wholewheat bread, tossed salad	grilled fish, mashed potatoes, steamed carrots, wholewheat roll, tea	beef broth, potato omelette, green salad, tea
snack	fruit salad with almonds and raisins	fruit yogurt	plain yogurt	crackers, tea

for several hours, generally about half a day, or two to three skipped meals. Once used up, and if food does not enter the body, protein from muscle and fat will be broken down and turned to glucose as energy.

With prolonged fasting, a physical state known as ketosis kicks in. Fasting causes water loss and large amounts of muscle breakdown because it is largely composed of protein. As muscle is broken down, nitrogen is eliminated from the body. Important minerals such as sodium, potassium and calcium are depleted and this has harmful effects on the body. Low potassium levels, for example, negatively affect the state of the heart and can even be a cause of death during fasting.

The kidneys have to work hard to get rid of the excess waste products with significant water loss. It is vital to drink lots of water during a total fast to avoid toxins accumulating in the blood and promote their elimination through urine. Although some people regard fasting as a detox method, be aware of the increase in waste products in the blood and other systems as byproducts of protein and fat breakdown. Fasting may give the intestinal tract a rest but the kidneys are overworked and other organs will suffer breakdown for use as energy.

The importance of glucose in a healthy functioning body cannot be overstated. The brain consumes the largest amount of glucose, so when blood sugar levels drop, the brain is unable to function properly. As a result, the person may feel confused, dizzy, lightheaded and have difficulty concentrating. The dieter may feel weak because the muscles are lacking in fuel and the blood is not pumping enough energy to the muscles and the cells. To make up for this decrease in energy, the metabolic rate slows down. Prolonged fasting is dangerous and not advised. In an attempt to moderate the physical consequences resulting from muscle loss, some variations

on the fasting method are more of a partial fast and include the consumption of juices.

Pros and cons
Weight loss results from fat and muscle being used up but also from any water loss. A quick way of shedding pounds, fasting is counter-productive to the body in the long term because once food is re-introduced, the body will gain weight quickly as it replenishes.

This all-or-nothing type of diet is not about moderation. After a period of deprivation, the dieter runs the risk either of eating uncontrollably or overeating.

Is it for you?
Fasting may appeal to someone who wants to lose weight quickly and is willing and able to undergo physical discomfort. A fast, however, should never exceed a period of two days. A complete lack of food will cause you to feel weak so restrict your activity levels.

Despite its popularity as a weight loss quick fix, fasting is generally not recommended by any dieticians. Patients with a heart condition or other illnesses should be very careful or avoid it altogether. Anyone considering going on a fast should consult a doctor before embarking on this extreme form of dieting.

Availability
The suggested food and drinks are widely available.

Lifestyle changes
None.

requires lots of fluids to eliminate waste products.

wednesday	thursday	friday
cold cereal, milk, banana, wholewheat toast and jam, tea	vanilla yogurt, honeydew, tea	tea and water throughout the day
vegetable stir fry with tofu, bok choy and peppers, brown rice, tea	vegetable soup, green salad, tea	tea and water throughout the day
beef barley soup, green salad, fruit salad, tea	miso soup, crackers, green tea	tea and water throughout the day
fruit and milk smoothie	cantaloupe, green tea	tea and water throughout the day

Resources
www.pccnaturalmarkets.com/health/
Diet/Fasting_Diet.htm

www.skinnyondiets.com/
TheFastingDiet.html

Adamson, E., Horning, L.
*The Complete Idiot's
Guide to Fasting*
(2002, Alpha Books)

Note: Fasts longer than one day are not recommended and should only be followed under medical supervision.

LONG-TERM PLAN

FLEXIBILITY

FAMILY FRIENDLY
●

COST
●●●

STRENGTH OF SCIENCE

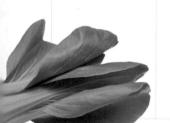

ROSEDALE DIET

High in healthy fats, this low-carbohydrate and moderate-protein diet is designed to control leptin levels, a hormone involved in weight loss and appetite.

Diet history
Created by metabolic specialist Ron Rosedale, MD, founder of the Rosedale Center in Denver, Colorado, and the Carolina Center for Metabolic Medicine in Asheville, North Carolina, who also published a book by the same name in 2004.

How does it work?
The diet's rationale is that because the hormone leptin plays a key role in the regulation of hunger, increasing the body's sensitivity to it can help to reduce cravings. Avoid most starchy carbs, sugars, saturated fats (in fatty meats or coconut) and trans fats (in non-dairy creams) but consume high quantities of healthy fats (in olive oil or rapeseed oil) and moderate amounts of proteins and high-fibre vegetables. Eat slowly and when hungry (rather than counting carbs or calories) and never less than three hours before going to bed. If hunger pangs are reduced, this can help to curb eating which promotes weight loss.

This high-fat, low-starch carb, moderate-to-low protein diet consists of two levels. Level One lasts 21 days and is the most restrictive on

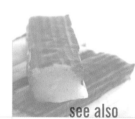

see also
atkins 42
south beach 64

sample menu
Level 1 is the most restrictive and offers fewer

	saturday	sunday	monday	tuesday
morning	hard-boiled eggs with pepper slices	scrambled eggs, turkey sausage	Omega-3 egg* omelette with spinach	smoothie with plain yogurt and 50g berries
lunch	poached salmon with pesto, salad greens	salad with walnuts and feta cheese	stir-fried chicken with broccoli and cashews	low-carb veggie burger, cucumber salad
supper	grilled mackerel, avocado slices	roast chicken, artichoke hearts, olive oil dipping sauce	grilled halibut with collard greens	grilled prawns with roasted red pepper and bok choy
snack 1	prawn dip, pepper strips	olive spread, crudités	olives, feta cheese	broccoli, hummus dip
snack 2	macadamia nuts	walnuts	almond butter, celery sticks	almonds

carbohydrate intake. Level Two is more relaxed but still somewhat rigorous about carbohydrate and protein consumption. It is also advisable to take multiple supplements throughout.

The scientifc evidence has confirmed the role of leptin in hunger regulation but there is little evidence to confirm both its contribution to actual weight loss or the need for taking the many supplements encouraged by the diet.

Pros and cons

In the Rosedale Diet, the dieter feels fuller for longer because of the kinds of foods included in the plan – those high in healthy fats such as fatty fish and nuts. High-fibre vegetables are encouraged at every meal which is also beneficial. The programme, however, may rate low in terms of the proteins and carbohydrates required by the body as nutrients. Some vitamin-rich fruit and vegetables such as pumpkin and grapes, for example, are entirely banned. Over 17 daily supplements are required which may prove expensive for some people.

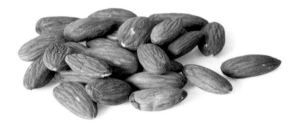

Is it for you?

With no calories to count or carbohydrate amounts to measure, the plan may appeal to individuals who like to eat when hungry and to those who prefer having lists of foods to tell them what they can or cannot have. Anyone on medication for a medical condition should check with their doctor or pharmacist before taking any of the supplements. With protein restricted to 50–80g a day, the Rosedale Diet may not be appropriate for most men or anyone who engages in vigorous physical activity and weight training.

Availability

All of the foods in this diet can be readily purchased from any general food shop or supermarket. The required multiple supplements can be bought from most manufacturers or directly from the author.

Lifestyle changes

Although not integral to the plan, exercise works as a good stress buster.

forbidden foods

- fried foods
- milk
- chickpeas
- sweetcorn
- pumpkin
- bananas
- oranges
- grapes

free foods

- almonds
- olives
- avocados
- fish and seafood
- tofu (soya beancurd)
- green, leafy vegetables
- skinless poultry
- mushrooms
- courgettes

carbohydrate options.

wednesday	thursday	friday
poached eggs with tomato and ham	grilled salmon with avocado	smoothie with pistachios
tuna salad with lettuce, olive oil vinaigrette	chicken on low-carb wrap with olive spread	antipasto salad, olive oil vinaigrette
grilled steak with roasted asparagus	prawn and scallop stir-fry with bamboo shoots	grilled white fish with roasted pepper sauce, broccoli
olives with Parmesan cubes	guacamole, raw carrots	pesto dip, crudités
pistachios	cashews	mixed nuts

Resources

Rosedale, R., Colman, C. *The Rosedale Diet* (2004, Harper Resource)

*Chicken eggs high in Omega-3 fats.

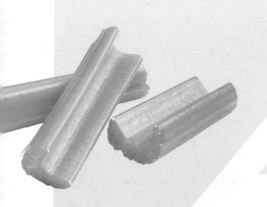

HEALTH-

This section discusses a variety of common diets that are used to promote well-being or manage specific health-related conditions. Hopefully, such diets **maximize health** status and **prevent one or a variety of illnesses** or disease conditions. For example, diets high in **whole grains, fibre, fruits and vegetables** are encouraged because they have been associated with a lowered risk of developing certain types of cancers. A variety of **low-fat diets** have been promoted for many years for decreasing the risk of heart disease. In efforts to promote the health of populations and decrease their risk of chronic disease, many food guides have also been developed. This section also includes some common **cultural food guides** that have become popular in promoting health – for example, the Mediterranean Diet Pyramid, the US MyPyramid, the Asian Diet Pyramid and the Latin American Diet Pyramid.

PROMOTION/
DISEASE-MANAGEMENT
PLANS

Conditions that may be treated by diet include allergies and intolerances, gastrointestinal disorders, problems related to carbohydrate utilization, heart disease and cancer. The diets may be prescribed by a doctor or registered dietician and used in a hospital or clinic setting to help treat disease, but those with chronic conditions usually need to learn and apply the eating guidelines to their everyday life to manage their disease and decrease the risk for complications. This is especially important with conditions such as diabetes, heart disease and hypertension.

The use of diets to treat disease is commonly referred to as Medical Nutrition Therapy (an older term is Diet Therapy). They are usually prescribed by a medical doctor and the instruction for the diet is given by a dietician. With a medical condition, it is important to consult a doctor before initiating any type of special diet and to do so with the advice of a practitioner who has extensive education in medical nutritional therapy, such as a registered dietician. Also, to check for possible contraindications, the healthcare professionals must be informed of any over-the-counter commercial formulas, special foods, herbals and supplements that are being used.

It is important to drink at least eight glasses of water per day.

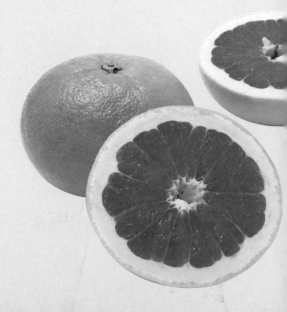

LONG-TERM PLAN

FLEXIBILITY

FAMILY FRIENDLY

COST

STRENGTH OF SCIENCE

ADDITIVE-FREE DIET

This meal plan excludes food additives – depending on individual tolerance, or preference, one or more additives may be eliminated.

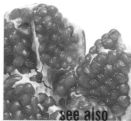

Diet history

One of the most popular additive-free diets is the Feingold Program. Dr Ben Feingold, a pediatrician who specialized in allergies, theorized that children are born with an inherited predisposition towards hyperactivity, which can be essentially or almost eliminated by following an additive-free diet. However, over the years, clinical studies have shown mixed results. An additive-free diet that eliminates either one or more food additives may also be used in the treatment of an allergy or intolerance to an additive.

How does it work?

A food additive is any substance that is added to food. Legal definitions vary by country. In the UK, an additive is considered a substance that affects the characteristics of a food. This includes substances used during production, processing, treatment, packaging, transportation or storage. Examples of long-established additives

see also
elimination 140

sample menu

Additive-free menus are based on the inclusion

	saturday	sunday	monday	tuesday
morning	freshly squeezed grapefruit juice, French toast, butter and honey	freshly squeezed orange juice, vegetable omelette, toast	freshly squeezed juice, scrambled eggs, homemade bread/toast	freshly squeezed orange juice, homemade blueberry muffin
lunch	pitta bread, homemade hummus, fresh fruit cup, milk	turkey sandwich, salad, milk	plain chicken breast, plain rice, steamed fresh carrots, milk	burger (100% beef), fresh pineapple, milk
supper	baked chicken, plain steamed fresh mixed vegetables, fresh peach, homemade mashed potatoes, milk	beef stir-fry with fresh vegetables, soya sauce, plain rice, fresh honeydew, milk	beef patty, steamed fresh asparagus, plain brown rice, milk	baked turkey, plain, steamed fresh green, beans, baked potato with butter, fresh cantaloupe, milk
snack 1	homemade muffin	fresh orange	celery sticks with peanut butter	plain low-fat yogurt
snack 2	plain yogurt with strawberries	corn chips and salsa	fresh raspberries	kiwi fruit

include salt, herbs and spices, sugar, and vinegar. Categories of additives include direct additives (such as artificial sweeteners), indirect additives (such as packaging substances) and colour additives.

The five main reasons for using additives are:
1 to maintain product consistency
2 to improve or maintain nutritional value
3 to maintain palatability and wholesomeness
4 to provide leavening or control acidity/alkalinity
5 to enhance flavour or impart colour.

While additive-free diets are often used in the treatment of conditions such as hyperactivity and attention deficit hyperactivity disorder (ADHD), the scientific literature is inconclusive to support their effectiveness. However, evidence strongly supports the use of an additive-free diet for the treatment of a true food allergy or intolerance to a specific additive.

Pros and cons
When used for treating food allergy, elimination of the additive may help relieve symptoms. Many foods marketed as additive-free (and there is a wide range of them) are healthy and nutrient rich.

weigh this up...
- Before beginning an additive-free diet, you should check with your doctor to ensure that the symptoms they are trying to eliminate are not caused by something other than a food additive.
- Eliminating multiple food additives at one time, especially in children, may also restrict food selection, and, ultimately, calorie intake, therefore a specialist should be consulted.
- Often, organic products are additive-free (check labels).
- Check meat for fillers and avoid those with additives.

The difficulties are that beginning a meal plan, like the Feingold Program, can be calorie and nutrient restricted, and food selection is reduced, especially with fruits and vegetables. Also, some of the products marketed as additive-free are expensive.

Is it for you?
Individuals suffering from unexplained allergy symptoms, which are not relieved by the removal of a single food, may want to consult a doctor or dietician about trying an additive-free diet.

Anyone trying to follow a more restricted additive-free meal plan, rather than just eliminating one or two additives, should consult a doctor and a registered dietician prior to beginning the programme. This is especially important for children, adolescents, pregnant or breastfeeding women, and the elderly.

Availability
Many of the foods have to be ordered or purchased at a speciality food shop.

Lifestyle changes
Learning which foods contain the food additive may take time. If multiple food additives are eliminated, dining out may be unrealistic.

of fresh homemade foods.

wednesday	thursday	friday
freshly squeezed grapefruit juice, hard-boiled egg, toast	freshly squeezed juice, bagel, peanut butter	freshly squeezed orange juice, cereal, milk
spinach salad with walnuts, fresh strawberries, homemade soup, milk	roast beef sandwich, homemade vegetable soup, milk	peanut butter and honey sandwich, homemade soup, milk
grilled steak, steamed cauliflower, baked sweet potato with cinnamon butter, fresh watermelon, milk	spaghetti with homemade sauce, steamed fresh broccoli, fresh plum, milk	baked veal, brown rice, steamed fresh carrots, fresh grapes, milk
pomegranate	avocado with lemon juice	fresh mango
fresh pineapple and cottage cheese	fresh blackberries	courgette sticks with homemade hummus

Resources

www.foodallergy.org

www.feingold.org

www.aaaai.org

Feingold, B., Feingold, H. *The Feingold Cookbook for Hyperactive Children* (1979, Random House)

Florida Dietic Association *Florida Manual of Medical Nutrition Therapy* (2007)

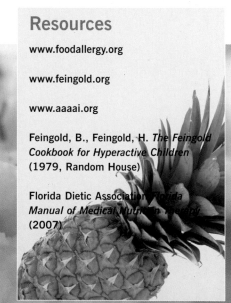

Note: This meal plan is from a general additive-free diet and not specifically the Feingold Program. Speciality products can be ordered to increase selection. All bought products, such as breads, cereals, tortilla chips, soya sauce and peanut butter, must be free of preservatives. Always check the labels.

LONG-TERM PLAN

FLEXIBILITY

FAMILY FRIENDLY

COST

STRENGTH OF SCIENCE

ASIAN DIET PYRAMID

This is a cultural model for healthy eating based on a diet high in fruit and vegetables and low in fat and cholesterol.

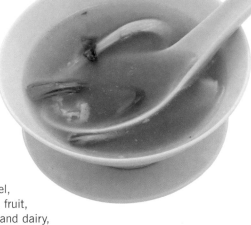

Diet history
Far Eastern (or Oriental) diets became popular because research showed that people who eat a plant-based diet show less risk of developing chronic diseases such as cancer, diabetes and heart trouble. The plant-based diet is partly responsible for the benefits. In 1992, Cornell University and the Harvard School of Public Health, along with the Oldways Preservation & Exchange Trust, developed the Asian Diet Pyramid model, which included a high consumption of grains, fruit, legumes and vegetables, low intakes of meat and dairy, with tea and other beverages.

How does it work?
This popular guide to help the population to stay healthy is based on the historical diets of rural Japan, China and other Far Eastern nations. Variations of the Asian food guide all have the same key

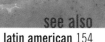

see also
latin american 154
mediterranean 160

sample menu

This healthy plan includes daily servings of green

	saturday	sunday	monday	tuesday
morning	sweet bean-filled steamed bun, kumquat and lychee salad, soya milk	cooked rice, poached egg, soya milk, pineapple juice	miso soup, soya milk, orange slices	corn meal made with soya milk, red grapes, black tea
lunch	ginger-marinated tofu steak, mange-tout with macadamia nuts, rice with bok choy, black tea	miso soup, spinach dumplings, fried rice with tofu, carrots, mange-tout and asparagus, ginger tea	buckwheat noodles with peanut sauce, shredded bok choy and cabbage with lime dressing, ginger tea	tofu salad with mixed greens, Korean-style cucumber pickles, lemon tea, pineapple chunks
supper	stir-fried pork strips, asparagus and spring onions, daikon salad, brown rice, sake	melon soup, mung bean noodles with cashews and mixed vegetables, black tea	bitter melon soup, grilled fish, brown rice, steamed broccoli, green tea	Thai-style noodles with peanuts and basil, steamed broccoli and cauliflower, soya milk
snack 1	cashews	fresh papaya slices	peanuts	watermelon
snack 2	fresh fruit salad	peanuts	pear	rice cake

elements – an eating plan high in fibre, vitamins and antioxidants due to the large proportion of fruit, legumes (such as soya) and vegetables, but low in meat, eggs, dairy products, saturated fats and cholesterol. Fish, tea and wine are allowed in moderate amounts. The diet is complemented by physical activity.

The diet's four categories are based on whether the foods are to be consumed daily, weekly, monthly or optionally. There are no serving sizes or number of servings per day, but the diet emphasizes adequacy and balance. The foods that can be eaten daily include green tea, grains, breads, vegetables, fruit, nuts, legumes, wine, beer and vegetable oils. The foods that can be consumed weekly include sweets (preferably fresh-fruit desserts), eggs and poultry. The foods that can be eaten monthly include red meat. Fish and shellfish, for example, are categorized as optional foods.

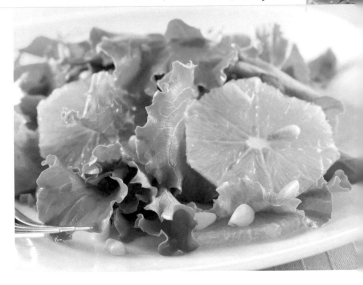

Pros and cons

All the varied foods in this diet are easy to prepare. Processed foods are kept down to a minimum and Oriental ingredients are colourful and appealing. The consumption of fruit, vegetables, soya beans and green tea can provide protection from cancer, obesity, heart disease and diabetes. The low consumption of dairy products, however, means that the diet may be deficient in calcium if calcium-rich vegetables are not eaten in sufficient quantities.

Is it for you?

The Asian Diet Pyramid is suitable for all healthy adults. A version for children has also now been developed.

Availability

The rice, fruit, vegetables, legumes and oils recommended in this diet are readily available from a specialist food shop or large supermarket.

Lifestyle changes

A low consumption of red meat and dairy products is part of the plan and a daily exercise programme is recommended.

tea, grains and nuts.

wednesday	thursday	friday
steamed noodles, green tea, plum compote	steamed spinach bun, strawberries, soya milk	vegetarian spring roll, pomelo, black tea
lemongrass chicken, brown rice with peas and spring onions, stir-fry vegetables, soya milk	tofu salad with ginger dressing, steamed aubergine with garlic sauce, brown rice, black tea	hot-and-sour soup with tofu, steamed millet with vegetables, broccoli with oyster sauce, black tea
tofu, spring onions, mushrooms, Swiss chard and daikon stir-fry, white rice, mango drink	prawns, bean sprouts, mange-tout and spring onion stir-fry, noodles, steamed carrots, orange tea	spicy lemon tofu with cashews, green salad with orange slices, sesame ginger dressing, soya milk
soya nuts	watermelon	edamame
mixed melon salad	sweet rice with mango	almond cookie

Resources

www.news.cornell.edu/chronicle/96/1.18.96/AsianDiet.html

www.oldwayspt.org/asian_pyramid.html

www.asiandiets.com

www.mediterrasian.com

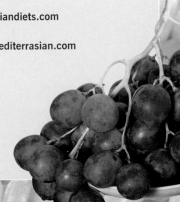

LONG-TERM PLAN

FLEXIBILITY

FAMILY FRIENDLY

COST

STRENGTH OF SCIENCE

CANDIDA DIET

This health-promotion strategy addresses the unhealthy balance of gastrointestinal yeast and bacteria that causes thrush by reducing yeast-forming foods in diet.

Diet history

The Candida Diet was developed in the 1980s by Dr William G. Crook, the man responsible for introducing the "yeast connection" in his book by the same name. Additional publications include *The Yeast Connection* (1986) and *Women's Health* (2003). The basis for his concept is the hypothesis that the overproduction of yeast in women is associated with the intake of yeast-forming foods and that certain chronic health-related problems may be reduced if these foods are avoided. Described in *The Yeast Connection*, the Candida Diet has been used and modified since its origination. Multiple variations of it are still being used and promoted today.

How does it work?

The plan's basis is the theory that an overabundance of the fungal organism *Candida Albicans* causes many chronic health problems in women such as chronic fatigue syndrome, sinusitis, irritable bowel syndrome, migraines and premenstrual syndrome (PMS). The goal is to help alleviate these complaints by creating a physiological balance of healthy bacteria and fungi in the intestinal tract, partly by the avoidance of those foods that are thought to cause fungal growth.

The diet eliminates all sugar (and foods containing sugar), simple carbohydrates, many fruits and pre-packed or processed foods due to

sample menu This plan is high in meat and vegetables, low in

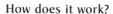

	saturday	sunday	monday	tuesday
morning	cooked quinoa, baked sweet potato, pecans	porridge, bacon, cashews	porridge with butter, water	brown rice with hazelnuts, sardines and rice cakes
lunch	egg, tuna or chicken salad with soya mayonnaise and tomato	hamburger patty, lettuce, tomato, onions	cos lettuce wrap with turkey and carrots, water	Caesar salad with grilled chicken breast, small amount of lemon juice
supper	tuna, broccoli, black-eyed peas	lamb chops, spinach salad with lemon juice, broccoli	baked chicken, steamed vegetables and pecans	hamburger patty, aubergine, mixed green salad

the additives and products they contain. To follow the diet, yeast-containing foods – including breads, dairy products, condiments, processed meats, malt products, most fruit and leftovers (due to the potential for mold formation) – must be strictly avoided for the first ten days of the programme.

The diet encourages the consumption of eight glasses of water per day but warns that tap water may contain unwanted lead, bacteria or parasites. Fruit juice, coffee, alcohol and diet drinks are not recommended either.

Some elements of the plan are used to treat certain types of yeast infections but data show that probiotics or yogurt are effective in enhancing the natural balance of bacteria and fungi present in the gastrointestinal tract. The Candida Diet per se does not provide the rationale as to why removal of certain foods (such as fruits, milk and breads) would accomplish this.

Pros and cons

The plan is very restrictive and eliminates essential nutrients such as calcium and B and C vitamins. Dieters may also find adhering to the programme challenging due to the removal of all "sugar-producing" items listed in the book, including processed products.

Is it for you?

The Candida Diet is likely to appeal to individuals who prefer a diet high in meat and vegetables but low in dairy and breads. The programme will be of interest to those suffering from chronic health problems (such as chronic fatigue and irritable bowel syndromes, migraine headaches or chronic sinusitis) who have not found other options helpful and are willing to adhere to the diet, or anyone who wants to reduce the presence of processed foods in their diet. There is little support for the idea that diet influences yeast content in the gastrointestinal tract.

Individuals should consult their doctor to determine if following the Candida Diet for a brief period of time may reduce or alleviate their chronic symptoms. A medical consultation is important, especially for individuals with pre-existing medical conditions.

Availability

The foods in this diet can be purchased from any general food shop or supermarket, but grocery shopping will involve careful label reading.

Lifestyle changes

Daily exercise and a sufficient water intake are recommended.

forbidden foods

- sugar
- fruit
- bread
- cheese
- milk
- fruit juice
- coffee
- diet drinks

treats

PICK FROM:
- beef
- chicken
- eggs
- fish
- nuts
- vegetables

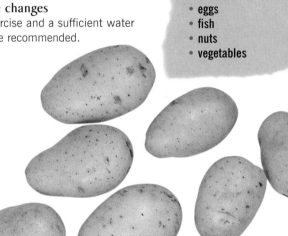

dairy and breads.

wednesday	thursday	friday
eggs, bacon, grits with butter	porridge, pork chops, cashew nuts	cooked amaranth, tuna, tomatoes, walnuts
vegetable salad with turkey strips on bed of cos lettuce	unsweetened yogurt and nuts	hard-boiled eggs, carrot and celery sticks
pork chops, turnip greens, okra, carrots, celery sticks	roast turkey, baked acorn squash, steamed spinach, cabbage and almonds, lemon juice, flaxseed oil dressing	cooked mixed vegetables and pecans

Resources

www.yeastconnection.com

Crook, W. G. *The Yeast Connection and Women* (1998, Professional Books)

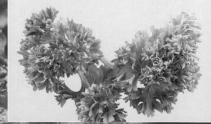

LONG-TERM PLAN
●●●

FLEXIBILITY
●●●

FAMILY FRIENDLY
●●●

COST
●

STRENGTH OF SCIENCE
●●●

DASH

Dietary Approaches to Stop Hypertension (DASH), designed to prevent and treat hypertension, is also used to reduce the risk of other chronic diseases, and is thus also called "the diet for all diseases".

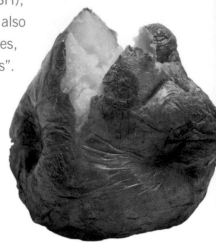

Diet history
This diet was developed for, and is based on, several large studies. The DASH Diet was first published by the National Heart Lung and Blood Institute of the National Institutes of Health, Department of Health and Human Services in 1998. It was revised in April 2006.

How does it work?
The diet was substantiated by several important studies, including Dietary Approaches to Stop Hypertension. This study, and others since, found that the less sodium consumed (1,500 mg), the greater the drop in blood pressure. The original diet used in the first study was 2,000 calories, low sodium (2,400 mg), high in mineral-rich fresh fruits and vegetables, and low in red meat (which reduced the intake of saturated fats and cholesterol, thereby reducing plaque accumulation in blood vessels). This combination diminished blood pressure levels in most participants but had the greatest effect

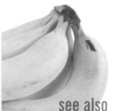

see also
low-sodium 156
mediterranean 160
tlc 176

sample menu
This plan emphasizes a plant-based diet, smaller

	saturday	sunday	monday	tuesday	
morning	low-fat muesli bar, banana, 100g yogurt, juice, milk	100g porridge, banana, milk, yogurt	juice, 40g cereal, milk, banana, bread, 1 tsp margarine	100g porridge, mini bagel, 1 tbsp peanut butter, banana, milk	
lunch	80g turkey, 2 slices bread, 1 slice cheese, lettuce or tomato, 1 tbsp mayonnaise, broccoli, orange	100g tuna, 1 tbsp mayonnaise, lettuce or tomato, 2 slices bread, apple, milk	80g chicken salad, 2 slices bread, salad, 1 tsp dressing, 70g fruit	80g chicken, 2 slices bread, 1 slice cheese, lettuce or tomato, 1 tbsp mayonnaise, cantaloupe, juice	
supper	80g fish (cooked with spices), 200g rice, sautéed spinach, roll, 1 tsp margarine, small biscuit	courgette lasagne, spinach salad, 1 tsp dressing, roll, 1 tsp margarine, juice	80g lean beef, baked potato, sour cream, roll, 1 tsp margarine, apple, milk	75g spaghetti, vegetable pasta sauce, spinach salad, 1 tsp dressing, 70g sweet corn, 70g pears	
snack 1	2 tbsp peanuts, milk	50g unsalted almonds, 40g dried apricots	50g unsalted almonds, 40g raisins	50g unsalted almonds, 40g dried apricots	
snack 2	40g dried apricots	6 crackers	100g yogurt	yogurt	

healthy tips

• At 1,600 calories, sweets are not included. At other calorie levels, the DASH is reduced in lean red meat, sweets, added sugars, and sugar-containing beverages compared to the typical Western diet.

Is it for you?
Those who have been diagnosed with high blood pressure may be more motivated to try the diet, especially if their healthcare provider recommends the plan. People with kidney disease may not be able to tolerate the high potassium content of the diet.

Availability
All the foods included in this diet are readily available from a grocery shop or supermarket.

on those with high blood pressure. Participants lost weight within days because they shed a lot of water-weight initially and within two weeks their blood pressure was significantly lower. Several calorie levels are now offered in the DASH diet, including 1,600 calories, 2,000 calories, 2,600 calories and 3,100 calories. The diet is recommended by health professionals for hypertension, weight loss and other chronic diseases, such as heart disease and metabolic syndrome.

Lifestyle changes
It is recommended to do 30 minutes per day of moderate exercise.

Pros and cons
The diet is low in saturated fat, cholesterol and total fat. It emphasizes fruits, vegetables and fat-free or low-fat milk and milk products, and includes whole grains, fish, poultry and nuts. It is also supported by extensive scientific research. The only disadvantage may be for those who have difficulty limiting red meat consumption and sugar consumption.

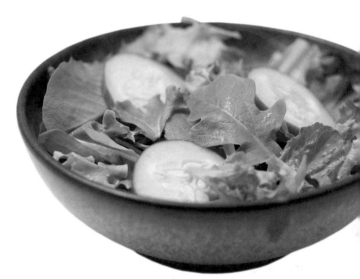

portions of lean meats and low-fat dairy.

wednesday	thursday	friday
80g puffed wheat, banana, milk, bread, 1 tsp margarine, juice	bread, yogurt, peach, 120ml juice	frosted shredded wheat, banana, milk, raisin bagel, 1 tbsp peanut butter, juice
55g beef, barbecue sauce, 2 slices cheese, bun, lettuce or tomato, potato salad, orange	55g ham, 1 slice cheese, 2 slices bread, lettuce or tomato, 1 tbsp mayonnaise, carrot sticks	100g tuna salad, 1 slice bread, cucumber or tomato salad, 110g cottage cheese, 70g pineapple, 1 tbsp almonds
80g fish, 100g brown rice, spinach, cornbread muffin	80g chicken Spanish rice, green peas, 140g cantaloupe, milk	80g turkey meatloaf, baked potato, sour cream, spring greens, roll, peach
2 crackers, 1 tbsp peanut butter	30g unsalted almonds, 40g dried apricots	fruit
yogurt	milk	100g yogurt, 1 tbsp sunflower seeds

Resources
www.nhlbi.nih.gov/health/public/heart/hbp/dash/new_dash.pdf

http://eatright.org/cps/rde/xchg/ada/hs.xsl/home_4380_ENU_HTML.htm

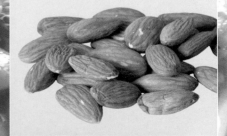

Note: All milk and milk products are fat free, low fat or skimmed; all margarine is low-fat tub or soft margarine; salad dressings and mayonnaise are all low fat; and all grain products are whole grain.

ELIMINATION DIET

LONG-TERM PLAN

FLEXIBILITY

FAMILY FRIENDLY
●

COST
●●

STRENGTH OF SCIENCE

The Elimination Diet is used for food allergies, including wheat, milk, egg, peanuts, soya, tree nuts, shellfish, fish and others.

Diet history

Adverse reactions to foods have been noted for over 2,000 years. Since the turn of the century, the medical literature has shown an increased interest in food reactions. It is believed that six to eight per cent of children develop food allergies within the first three years of life. Most children outgrow these allergies. In adults, the prevalence is estimated to be one to five per cent.

Diagnosis of food allergies is difficult due to varied diagnostic criteria. However, once a food allergy is diagnosed the main principle of dietary management is avoidance of the food that contains the proteins that cause the clinical symptoms.

How does it work?

Eight foods are thought to account for more than 90 per cent of all food allergies. These include eggs, milk, wheat, peanuts, soya, tree nuts, shellfish and fish.

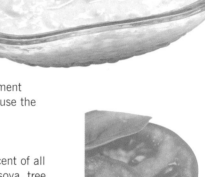

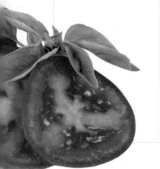

see also
additive-free 132

sample menu

One-day samples for each of the common allergies.

	egg allergy	milk allergy	wheat allergy	peanut allergy
morning	240ml juice, 100g porridge, 1 slice wholewheat bread, 1 tsp margarine, 240ml 1% milk	calcium-fortified orange juice, 50g cereal, 240ml soya milk, 1 slice ham, 1 tsp margarine, 1 slice toast	calcium-fortified orange juice, gluten-free waffles with margarine and 30g syrup, scrambled eggs	bread, 200g yogurt, peach, 120ml juice
lunch	80g chicken breast, baked potato with shredded cheese, 1 tsp margarine, sliced tomatoes, 140g strawberries	100g tuna salad, lettuce or tomato, 1 slice wheat bread, 240ml chicken vegetable soup, 80g broccoli, fresh fruit	2 slices gluten-free rice bread, sliced turkey, cheese slice, lettuce or tomato, baby carrots, red grapes	55g beef, 1 slice cheese, 2 slices bread, lettuce or tomato, 1 tbsp mayonnaise, 150g carrot sticks
supper	40g ham, 200g mashed potato, 80g broccoli, lettuce salad, 1 slice bread, 1 tsp margarine	80g roast beef, baked potato, 1 tsp margarine, spinach salad, 1 tbsp oil and vinegar dressing, 120g mixed fruit	80g salmon with lemon, sweet potato, 1 tsp margarine, broccoli with olive oil and garlic, mixed salad, 1 tbsp oil and vinegar dressing	80g chicken, Spanish rice, 200g green peas, 170g cantaloupe, 240ml milk
snack 1	200g plain low-fat yogurt	70g unsalted almonds, 40g dried apricots	30g plain almonds, 1 apple	40g dried apricots
snack 2	1 orange	1 cup yogurt	200g plain yogurt, 70g strawberries	240ml milk

An elimination diet is the only way to combat a food allergy. The principle is that if the offending food is removed from the diet, the food-induced illness will be resolved. Elimination diets, followed by the return of suspected foods to the diet, should be applied only in situations where allergy symptoms are not life threatening. Care must be taken that the suspected foods are not inadvertently consumed while hidden in other foods. People with allergies need nutrition counselling to help them know what to look for on food labels.

weigh this up...
• Simply avoiding the food that causes the reaction is not as simple as it sounds. For example, egg protein may be called albumin, egg white, egg yolk, globulin, ovalbumin, ovomucin, ovovitelin, Simplesse®, livetin or lecithin on a food label. Even egg substitutes often contain egg proteins.

Pros and cons
The Elimination Diet is effective in preventing food allergy symptoms. The disadvantage is that, depending on how many food allergies the person has, the diet can be very restrictive and could result in nutrient deficiencies. Learning the names of all possible food ingredients for each allergy, and obtaining ingredient lists for restaurant foods, may be difficult.

Is it for you?
This is suitable for people who have been diagnosed with specific food allergies and those with gastrointestinal disorders who want to track down the foods that contribute to the symptoms.

The diet can be very restrictive, so caution should be exercised to eliminate only the foods that contribute to symptoms.

Availability
Depending on the allergy, the diet foods are readily available but some must be ordered from specific producers or speciality suppliers.

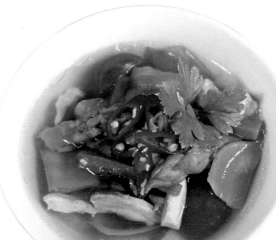

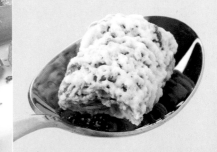

Gluten-free bread.

Lifestyle changes
None. This diet specifically addresses food restriction to alleviate symptoms.

soya allergy	tree-nut allergy	seafood allergy
50g frosted shredded wheat, banana, 240ml milk, raisin bagel, 1 tbsp peanut butter, 1 cup juice	50g corn flakes, banana, 100g plain yogurt, 240ml juice, 240ml milk	100g porridge, banana, milk, 100g yogurt
50g tuna salad, 2 slices bread, cucumber or tomato salad, 100g cottage cheese, 170g pineapple	80g turkey, 2 slices bread, 1 slice cheese, lettuce or tomato, 1 tbsp mayonnaise, 160g broccoli, orange	65g chicken, 1 tbsp mayonnaise, lettuce or tomato, 2 slices bread, apple, 240ml milk
80g turkey meatloaf, baked potato, sour cream, spring greens, roll, peach	80g grilled fish, 200g yellow rice, 200g spinach, roll, 1 tsp margarine, vanilla pudding	courgette lasagne, lettuce salad, 1 tsp dressing, roll, 1 tsp margarine, 240ml juice
fruit	240ml milk	50g unsalted almonds, 40g dried apricots
100g yogurt, 1 tbsp sunflower seeds	40g dried apricots	6 crackers

Resources
www.foodallergy.org

www.aafa.org

Reference: *Florida Manual of Medical Nutrition Therapy* (2007). Florida Dietetic Association, Tallahassee, FL.

LONG-TERM PLAN

FLEXIBILITY

FAMILY FRIENDLY

COST

STRENGTH OF SCIENCE

GERD DIET

This diet plan is designed for those who have gastro-oesophageal reflux disease. Dietary modifications are intended to help reduce the occurrence of reflux and minimize oesophageal irritation.

Diet history

Dietary treatment for GERD has a long medical history, including many variations, with the general focus tending to be on minimizing the symptoms. One of the most common symptoms is heartburn, which occurs as a result of stomach acid (with a pH close to battery acid) rising back into the oesophagus. This is due to the band of lower oesophageal sphincter (LOS) muscles not working properly. Usually, the LOS works like a rubber band between the stomach and the oesophagus. It prevents the stomach acid from coming back up. However, with GERD some of the acid does come back into the oesophagus, resulting in irritation.

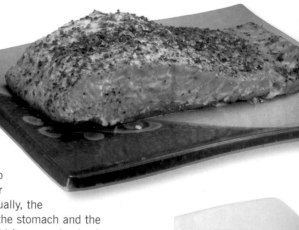

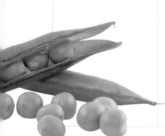

sample menu

In this menu high-fat foods, citrus foods, caffeine

	saturday	sunday	monday	tuesday
morning	porridge with cinnamon and raisins, hard-boiled egg, decaf hot tea (not mint)	wholegrain cereal with almonds (small amount), wholegrain toast, fresh watermelon, skimmed milk	wholegrain bagel, with margarine, egg substitute or egg white, plum slices, skimmed milk	porridge with walnuts added (small amount), fresh honeydew, 100% apple juice with added vitamin C
lunch	wholewheat pitta, hummus (homemade, low fat), mango slices, skimmed milk	tuna salad (water-packed tuna with fat-free mayo), wholegrain crackers, veggie sticks, skimmed milk	turkey sandwich on, wholegrain bread, chicken noodle soup, apple slices, skimmed milk	lean roast beef, sandwich on wholegrain bun, fresh fruit salad (no citrus), skimmed milk
supper	baked turkey, brown rice, steamed veggie mix, fresh pear slices, skimmed milk	baked ham, sugar snap peas, jasmine rice, fresh fruit cup (no citrus), skimmed milk	grilled salmon, steamed asparagus, brown rice, fresh blueberries, water	baked chicken, steamed green beans, baked potato with margarine, fresh cantaloupe, skimmed milk
snack 1	fat-free cottage cheese with berries	low-fat fruit smoothie	crackers	fat-free cottage cheese with peaches
snack 2	rice cake	sorbet or sherbet	fat-free yogurt	carrot sticks with fat-free dressing

How does it work?

The diet aims to help minimize reflux and irritation to the oesophagus. Large meals are discouraged because they increase stomach pressure and may increase reflux. The diet recommends eating no less than three hours prior to bedtime to avoid laying down following a meal. Reflux may be promoted by obesity. Achieving a healthy body weight is important. Decreasing calories promotes weight loss, if needed.

Chocolate should be avoided because it contains methylxanthine, which may relax the lower oesophageal sphincter. Fat may be restricted if high-fat foods tend to make the reflux worse. Some other foods and beverages to avoid include citrus fruits and juices, caffeinated beverages, carbonated beverages and coffee (caffeinated and decaffeinated). They can irritate an already inflamed lower oesophagus. Peppermint and spearmint may aggravate acid reflux and should be avoided. Nicotine weakens the lower oesophageal muscle, so smoking should be avoided.

Pros and cons

The foods and beverages are low in fat and all food groups are included in the meal plan. Consuming small meals and snacks during the day should promote a feeling of satiety, which is especially good if trying to lose weight.

However, eliminating treat foods, such as chocolate, and some beverages (coffee for example) may be difficult at first. Avoiding large meals, especially when dining out, may be challenging.

healthy tips
- Buy allowed juices that are fortified with vitamin C as citrus fruits and juices should be avoided.
- Consume lower-fat and fat-free dairy products for adequate calcium but without excess fat.
- Tolerance is unique to the individual. This plan is simply a guide to which foods and drinks can be added as they are tolerated (for example, coffee or tomatoes).

Is it for you?

This meal plan may suit someone who has GERD or reflux. It is healthy and appropriate for everyone if it is nutritionally well planned.

Availability

Most of the foods are easily accessible and available. There are a few speciality items.

Lifestyle changes

Changes include avoiding large meals, decreasing total fat intake, losing weight if necessary, avoiding coffee, avoiding chocolate, stopping smoking, and avoiding eating within three hours of bedtime.

and chocolate are eliminated.

wednesday	thursday	friday	**Resources**
wholewheat, pancakes with syrup, fresh raspberries, decaf hot tea (not mint)	veggie omelette (made with egg substitute), fresh blackberries, wholewheat toast, 100% grape juice	wholegrain scone with nut butter (small amount), fresh peach, skimmed milk	www.aboutgerd.org Magee, E. *Tell Me What to Eat If I Have Acid Reflux: Nutrition You Can Live With* (2002, The Career Press)
lean ham sandwich on wholegrain bread, garden salad with fat-free dressing, skimmed milk	grilled chicken sandwich on wheat bun, lentil soup, fresh melon cup, skimmed milk	veggie wrap, spinach salad with fat-free dressing, fresh strawberries, skimmed milk	
lean steak, steamed cauliflower, baked sweet potato, fresh berry cup, skimmed milk	grilled white fish, couscous, steamed fresh broccoli, fresh plum, skimmed milk	baked pork loin, mashed potatoes, steamed carrots, fresh grapes, skimmed milk	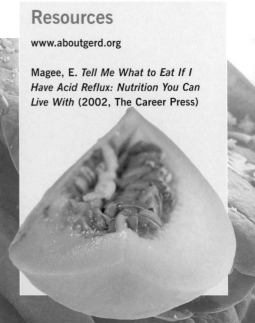
unsweetened apple sauce	apple slices with light-fat or fat-free cheese	celery and carrot sticks with fat-free dressing	
low-fat yogurt drink	pretzels	fresh fruit (no citrus)	

LONG-TERM PLAN
●●●

FLEXIBILITY
●●

FAMILY FRIENDLY
●●

COST
●

STRENGTH OF SCIENCE
●●●

GLUTEN-FREE DIET

Prescribed to gluten-intolerant individuals, this diet treats the digestive complaint triggered by intolerance to foods like wheat, barley and rye.

Diet history

First identified by the ancient Greek physician Aretaeus of Cappadocia, the history of coeliac disease dates back to around AD 250 but it was 1888 before British medical practitioner Dr Samuel Gee was able to document a therapy. The link with gluten was finally identified in 1952 when Dutch paediatrician Dr Willem Karel Dicke observed that the intolerance was caused by wheat proteins.

The status of the Gluten-Free Diet as a form of nutritional therapy was confirmed in 1954. This lifelong diet has become increasingly popular as the global prevalence of coeliac disease is currently estimated at one in every 266 people. The charity Coeliac UK estimates that one per cent of the UK population has the condition, many undiagnosed.

How does it work?

When a person suffers from coeliac disease (also known as coeliac sprue or gluten sensitive enteropathy), he or she develops an inability

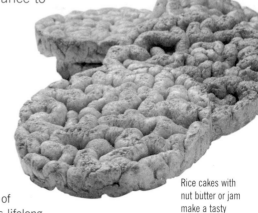

Rice cakes with nut butter or jam make a tasty snack.

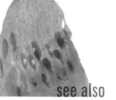

see also
elimination 140

sample menu

Product ingredients will vary so always read the

	saturday	sunday	monday	tuesday
morning	cream of buckwheat, orange slices, gluten-free toast with nut butter, hot tea (unflavoured)	hard-boiled egg, gluten-free toast, banana, calcium-fortified orange juice	gluten-free bagel with cream cheese, calcium-fortified orange juice, fresh blueberries	gluten-free waffle with syrup, thick-cut bacon, fresh honeydew, hot tea (unflavoured)
lunch	toasted cheese sandwich with gluten-free bread, tomato soup, apple slices, milk	turkey sandwich with gluten-free bread and gluten-free turkey, salad with gluten-free croutons, pineapple, milk	lentil soup, rice crackers, spinach salad with gluten-free croutons, milk	gluten-free veggie pizza, mixed fresh fruit cup topped with nuts, milk
supper	roast chicken, plain, steamed squash, onions and red peppers, mashed potatoes, peach, milk	gluten-free baked ham, steamed broccoli and cauliflower, jasmine rice, fresh melon cup, milk	gluten-free smoked salmon, steamed fresh asparagus, plain brown rice, milk	roast chicken, steamed green beans, baked potato with butter, fresh cantaloupe, milk
snacks	gluten-free muffin, trail mix with gluten-free muesli	rice cakes with nut butter, baked corn chips and salsa	celery sticks with peanut butter and raisins, fresh fruit	plain low-fat yogurt with fresh fruit, gluten-free snack bar

weigh this up...

- Commercially available oats or products containing oats are not recommended by coeliac organizations in the UK. Pure, uncontaminated speciality oat products are now available in most large shops and supermarkets, and some associations will allow moderate amounts.

to digest a form of protein in the diet called gluten. Sources include wheat, rye, barley and their respective by-products. Oats, too, may contain gluten if cross-contaminated. When gluten-rich foods are eaten by sufferers, their immune system produces gluten antibodies which cause the small intestinal tract where the absorption of nutrients such as calcium, iron and folate takes place to flatten and become inflamed. The Gluten-Free plan facilitates the absorption of these vital nutrients.

Pros and cons

The Gluten-Free Diet is effective as a treatment for coeliac disease and in recent years the variety and availability of gluten-free products has increased substantially. Certain speciality products, however, are still expensive and many foods today contain a wheat component to some degree or other, so grocery shopping requires a watchful eye when reading food labels. Dining out and takeaway menus can also be challenging if you are trying to trace the source of ingredients used.

Is it for you?

Coeliac disease sufferers need to follow this diet for life. Combined with a casein-free diet, the Gluten-Free Diet is now a popular treatment for individuals with autism. However, the scientific data remains inconclusive. If nutritionally well balanced, this plan is suitable for all.

Availability

Gluten-free products are now widely available both in grocery shops and via the Internet.

Lifestyle changes

Get ready to discover which ingredients to avoid, learn to read food labels and prepare gluten-free recipes, and locate restaurants offering gluten-free dishes on their menus.

foods allowed

- amaranth
- arrowroot
- buckwheat
- corn bran
- corn flour
- flax
- legume flours
- teff (gluten-free Ethiopian grain)
- tapioca
- cassava

forbidden foods

- wheat (including durum, kamut and spelt)
- barley (including beer, lager, malt, brewer's yeast)
- rye (including rye bread and flour)

labels carefully.

wednesday	thursday	friday
puffed corn cereal with milk, gluten-free toast with butter, kiwi fruit, hot tea (unflavoured)	cream of brown rice cereal, fresh strawberries, calcium-fortified orange juice	gluten-free bagel with scrambled eggs and cheese, calcium-fortified apple juice
ham sandwich with gluten-free bread, gluten-free ham and cheese, chicken and rice soup, milk	bean burrito made with corn tortilla, white rice, papaya, milk	low-fat cottage cheese and fruit plate, gluten-free cream of mushroom soup, milk
grilled gluten-free steak, steamed cauliflower, baked sweet potato with cinnamon and butter, watermelon, milk	gluten-free baked fish, gluten-free macaroni and cheese, steamed fresh broccoli, plums, milk	gluten-free pork loin, baked brown rice, steamed carrots, grapes, milk
plain popcorn, fresh fruit and low-fat cottage cheese	gluten-free soya nuts, rice crackers and cheese cubes	gluten-free pretzels, courgette sticks with hummus

Resources

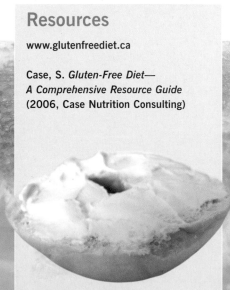

www.glutenfreediet.ca

Case, S. *Gluten-Free Diet— A Comprehensive Resource Guide* (2006, Case Nutrition Consulting)

Note: Prepare these gluten-free ingredients at home or buy commercially available gluten-free products.

LONG-TERM PLAN
●●●

FLEXIBILITY
●●

FAMILY FRIENDLY
●●●

COST
●

STRENGTH OF SCIENCE
●●●

GOOD MOOD DIET

Touted as the eating plan to end diet miseries, this two-stage plan incorporates wholesome foods, physical activity and positive attitude for healthy well-being.

Diet history
Written by Dr Susan Kleiner, RD, the Good Mood Diet is the result of over 25 years of providing nutrition counselling to a diverse range of clients, including professional athletes. The Good Mood diet has helped numerous citizens of Seattle lose weight through the highly publicized challenge in the Seattle Post-Intelligencer.

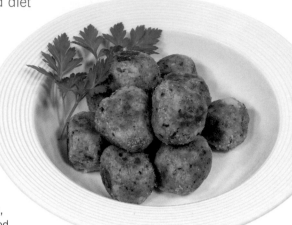

Baked salmon patties.

How does it work?
The rationale for the diet is that by choosing foods that are healthy and nutritious, along with plenty of rest and physical activity, optimal physical and emotional health can be achieved. Foods are classified as either "feel-great foods" or "feel-bad foods".

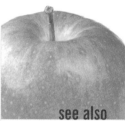

see also
intuitive eating 148
tlc 176

sample menu

This plan emphasizes healthy foods like fruits

	saturday	sunday	monday	tuesday
morning	wholewheat pancakes with flaxseed, fresh berries, soya sausage	egg-white omelette, wholewheat toast, orange	breakfast burrito with corn tortilla and salad, mango, skimmed milk	oat bran with flaxseed and berries, boiled egg, skimmed milk
lunch	turkey slices, tomato and cucumber salad, bean soup, water	tuna salad on spinach, small soup	wholewheat turkey sandwich, spinach salad, water	low-fat chicken salad on mixed greens, vegetable soup, water
supper	avocado slices, wholewheat fish tacos, orange, water	roast chicken, asparagus, roast red pepper and pumpkin with dates, brown rice	bean soup, grilled grouper, vegetable medley	fish tacos with grilled vegetables, clementine, water
snack 1	soya crackers	berries with yogurt	air-popped popcorn	apple and celery
snack 2	skimmed milk	edamame	low-fat hot chocolate	boiled egg

During the first two weeks of the programme, the Feel Good Accelerator, feel-bad foods are eliminated. Various calorie levels are provided, with food group servings for three meals and two snacks. During the second level, Feel Great While You Lose Weight Phase, two servings of wine, chocolate or added sugar may be re-introduced in moderation. Once weight-loss goals are achieved, diets are switched over into the Good Mood for a Lifetime.

The book provides many recipes and ideas, such as foods to carry for snacks, or how to choose the best options when eating on the go. This diet emphasizes choosing foods from the food groups that are highest in nutrients and stresses moderation and variety. It carries a holistic approach to nourishing the body and mind and is based on solid science-based principles.

Pros and cons
Both stages are healthy for long-term use. They allow flexibility in food choices while assisting with suggested food groups and portions. There are different calorie groups based on gender and activity. The disadvantage is that the approach may be too lenient for those who need more guidance.

weigh this up…
- Feel-bad foods include large quantities of alcohol and caffeine, fried foods, fatty meats, fatty snack foods, refined sugars, and starches.
- Feel-good foods include bananas, berries, cocoa powder, eggs, flaxseed, ginger, garlic, turkey, whole greens, dark green and orange vegetables, soya and tofu.

Is it for you?
This is ideal for those who are looking for more energy through diet and physical activity, and need direction in making healthy lifestyle changes.

This diet emphasizes choosing healthy foods in combination with physical activity. Unless there are specific health conditions that require a special diet, this plan has no restrictions.

Availability
All the foods in this diet can be bought in general food shops or supermarkets.

Lifestyle changes
The diet focuses on making the connection between diet, mood and physical activity. It recommends getting plenty of rest, becoming increasingly active and walking 10,000 steps daily with the use of a pedometer.

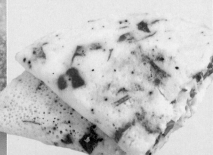

and lean meats for physical and mental well-being.

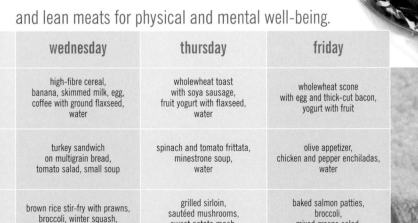

wednesday	thursday	friday
high-fibre cereal, banana, skimmed milk, egg, coffee with ground flaxseed, water	wholewheat toast with soya sausage, fruit yogurt with flaxseed, water	wholewheat scone with egg and thick-cut bacon, yogurt with fruit
turkey sandwich on multigrain bread, tomato salad, small soup	spinach and tomato frittata, minestrone soup, water	olive appetizer, chicken and pepper enchiladas, water
brown rice stir-fry with prawns, broccoli, winter squash, water	grilled sirloin, sautéed mushrooms, sweet potato mash, corn-on-the-cob	baked salmon patties, broccoli, mixed greens salad, orange
turkey slices	peanuts in shell	air-popped popcorn
smoothie	low-sodium vegetable juice	turkey jerky

Resources
www.goodmooddiet.com

www.powereating.com

Kleiner, S. *The Good Mood Diet* (2005, Springboard Press)

INTUITIVE EATING

Intuitive Eating is a plan that discourages dieting and emphasizes a positive approach to food. It is a process of re-learning to eat when hungry and not ignoring cravings.

LONG-TERM PLAN

FLEXIBILITY

FAMILY FRIENDLY

COST
●

STRENGTH OF SCIENCE

Diet history
Written by Evelyn Tribole, RD, and Elyse Resch, RD, this approach is based on their experiences in helping clients create a healthy relationship with their food, mind and body. In its second edition, the book claims to be "a revolutionary programme that works".

How does it work?
The rationale behind the plan is that diets cause more harm than good. The authors propose that dieting leads to deprivation, food obsessions, cravings, binges and may lead to disordered eating.

Based on ten principles, individuals are guided to reject the dieting mentality, honour hunger, make peace with food, challenge negative internal voices, understand and discover hunger and satisfaction, cope with emotional food issues, respect the body, be physically active and honour nutrition and health.

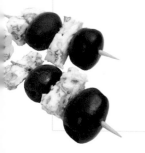

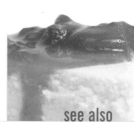

see also
good mood 146
overeaters anonymous 166

sample menu
This plan rejects the diet mentality and encourages

	saturday	sunday	monday	tuesday
morning	pancakes, syrup, scrambled eggs, orange slices, coffee	porridge with raspberries, wholewheat toast, jam, grapefruit, milk, coffee	cereal with skimmed milk, banana, peanut butter, coffee	porridge with berries, toast with cheese, chocolate milk
lunch	turkey and Swiss cheese on rye bread, fresh berries with yogurt, tomato slices with oil and vinegar	junior cheeseburger with small fries, diet soft drink, apple	vegetable soup, turkey sandwich, yogurt	tuna salad sandwich, pudding, carrot sticks
supper	baked beans, grilled chicken breast, corn-on-the-cob, peach with light whipped cream	mixed greens with spinach salad, black beans, brown rice, avocado slices, broccoli	wholewheat pasta with sauce, salmon, spinach, salad	brown rice, sweet potato, Brussels sprouts, chicken
snack 1	olives with cheese	cantaloupe and yogurt	2 biscuits	3 chocolates
snack 2	glass of red wine	popcorn	apple	low-fat cheese

The ultimate goal is to feel comfortable with eating without the dieting mentality and therefore the plan does not include a "diet" to follow. Through exercising for fun and making intuitive choices, weight loss occurs naturally. The plan is based on solid principles and has had positive results in various research studies.

Pros and cons

This outlook emphasizes the process of learning to listen to our bodies for hunger cues and using good nutrition knowledge for choosing foods. It also allows for flexibility in selecting snacks and foods.

However, the disadvantage is that the process may be too long for persons who have been conditioned to the dieting mentality. Some may require professional counselling to work through their emotions and relationships to food.

Is it for you?

This diet is likely to appeal to those who have struggled with diets and weight for years and need to develop a healthy relationship with food and their bodies. The plan emphasizes developing a healthy relationship between emotions and food. Anyone can follow this plan. However, individuals with health conditions may need to follow specialized diets.

Availability

The foods can be bought in any larger supermarkets.

Lifestyle changes

The book emphasizes the importance of physical activity as an energy and mood booster. It encourages exercise as a way to care for yourself and not to focus on the weight-loss component.

weigh this up...

- Eliminate Destructive Voices, Beware of the Food Police, the Nutrition Informant, and the Diet Rebel Voices! The Food Police voice scrutinizes our every bite and keeps us at war with food, while the Nutrition Informant voice unconsciously promotes dieting with an authoritarian voice. The Diet Rebel voice screams determined to rebel against dieting.
- Listen for Your Powerful Ally Voices Develop skills to hear the Food Anthropologist, the Nurturer, the Nutrition Ally and the Rebel Ally Voices! These voices are neutral and gentle when working through the plan's ten steps. They allow the individual to set boundaries and make healthy choices without guilt. They are effective voices in combating negative self-talk.

treats to satisy cravings.

	wednesday	thursday	friday
	omelette with spinach and turkey sausage, orange juice, coffee	low-fat cheese, egg and thick-cut bacon on a muffin, banana, coffee	cereal with raisins, skimmed milk, boiled egg
	mixed greens salad with chickpeas and beetroot, cottage cheese, wholewheat roll	vegetarian burger on wholewheat bun, oven chips, broccoli	lentil soup, wholewheat baguette, spinach salad
	vegetable lasagne, asparagus, garden salad with tomato, sliver of chocolate cake	bean enchiladas, beetroot salad, green beans	Chinese vegetable stir-fry with wholewheat noodles, 2 fried wontons, skimmed milk
	glass of wine, cheese, apple	low-fat yogurt	1 small slice cheesecake
	carrots with low-fat dressing	fruit salad	blueberries

Resources

www.intuitiveeating.com

http://health.dailynewscentral.com/content/view/0001939/41/

Tribole, E., Resch, E. *Intuitive Eating* (2003, 2nd ed., St. Martin's Press)

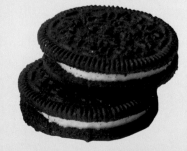

Note: This menu is in the style of MyPyramid using Intuitive Eating and taken from *Intuitive Eating*.

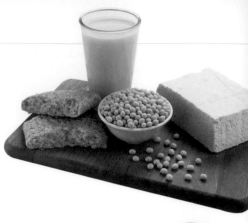

LONG-TERM PLAN
●●●

FLEXIBILITY
●●●

FAMILY FRIENDLY
●●●

COST
●

STRENGTH OF SCIENCE
●●●

LACTO-OVO VEGETARIAN DIET

This plan excludes meat, poultry, and fish but includes fruit, vegetables, grains, nuts, seeds, dairy products and eggs.

Diet history
The first vegetarian diet originated around the first millennium BC. Non-meat eaters were called Pythagoreans after Pythagoras, the Greek philosopher and mathematician. The term "vegetarian", however, did not exist before 1847. Although global estimates are not available, a 2004 Food Standards Agency survey revealed that five per cent of UK households claimed to have at least one vegetarian member.

How does it work?
The Lacto-Ovo Vegetarian diet includes fruit, vegetables, seeds, nuts, grains, legumes, dairy (lacto) and eggs (ovo). Eggs and dairy and soya products provide high-quality protein as do other food combinations such as grains and legumes, or seeds and nuts (for example, a peanut butter sandwich). If nutritionally balanced, this plan is considered to be a healthy way of eating. This meal plan may help in the prevention of some cancers, maintaining a healthy heart, low blood pressure and weight management.

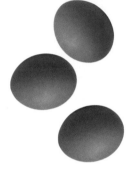

see also
vegan 178

sample menu
This menu includes meat substitutes such as

	saturday	sunday	monday	tuesday
morning	veggie bacon, wholegrain waffle with maple syrup, apple, grape juice	scrambled eggs, wholewheat toast, kiwi fruit, cranberry juice	wholewheat bagel, peanut butter, strawberries, orange juice	veggie omelette, wholewheat toast, banana, hot tea
lunch	soya hot dog in a wholewheat bun, vegetarian baked beans, apple sauce, milk	veggie pizza, garden salad, strawberries, milk	spinach salad with oranges, gorgonzola, walnuts, raspberry vinaigrette dressing, tomato bisque soup, wholewheat crackers, milk	tofu and veggie burrito, blue corn chips with salsa, pineapple, milk
supper	green pepper stuffed with rice and tofu crumble, carrots, wholewheat dinner roll, pear, milk	tofu and veggie kebabs, couscous, mango, milk	faux chicken patty, broccoli with red peppers and onions, wild rice with pecans and raisins, plums, milk	bean loaf, mashed cauliflower, steamed green beans with slivered almonds, wholewheat dinner roll, grapes, milk
snacks	wholewheat crackers, natural peanut butter	fruit smoothie (made with fresh fruit and yogurt)	yogurt with honey, peaches and granola	wholewheat pitta, hummus

weigh this up...
- Focus on getting enough high-quality protein, calcium, vitamins D and B12, zinc and iron.
- Foods full of vitamin C consumed alongside those rich in iron can triple the absorption of the kind of iron found in all plant-based foods. Complementary proteins, such as peanut butter and bread, do not have to be consumed at the same meal but need to be eaten within 24 hours.

Pros and cons

High-quality proteins contain all the amino acids essential for growth. Some foods can be combined to provide all the essential amino acids. Also, plant-based foods are less expensive than meat, an increased consumption of fruit and vegetables can help to prevent disease, and a greater intake of phytochemicals and fibre is nutritionally beneficial. The diet, however, needs to be planned carefully to meet all nutrient requirements.

Is it for you?

The vegetarian meal plan may appeal to individuals who are health and/or environmentally conscious. When not following this diet for weight-loss reasons, the foods specified can be eaten liberally. When following the diet for weight management, salads with fat-free dressing and non-starchy vegetables can be added to the meal plan to increase satiety without drastically increasing calories.

Carefully planned, the Lacto-Ovo Vegetarian Diet is appropriate for everyone. However, it is critical that the meal plan be evaluated as a satisfactory source of nutrients for pregnant and breastfeeding women, and for children and teenagers.

Availability

The foods and drinks in this diet are widely available as are meat substitutes and soya- or rice-based milks, cheese, yogurt and other products. Many restaurants and schools now offer vegetarian choices.

Lifestyle changes

Gradual behaviour modification is key when switching over to this diet. You will have to read all food labels, plus shop for and learn to prepare lacto-ovo vegetarian recipes. This takes time and practice. Education on the appropriate, nutrient-dense types of foods is also essential.

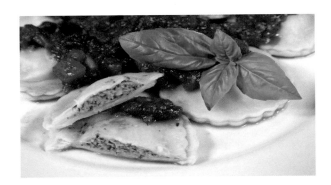

faux chicken patties (bought or homemade).

wednesday	thursday	friday
veggie sausage patty, multigrain scone, cantaloupe and honeydew cup, apple juice	porridge, hard-boiled egg, orange, hot tea	wholegrain cereal with soya milk, blueberries, cheese toast (with wholewheat bread and light cheese), orange juice
pimento cheese sandwich on wholegrain bread, lentil soup, fruit cup, milk	tofu reuben sandwich, baked sweet potato fries, raspberries and blueberries with fat-free whipped topping, milk	vegetarian chilli (made from soya), grilled cheese and tomato sandwich on wholewheat bread, carrot and courgette sticks with ranch dressing, peach slices topped with plain yogurt, milk
spinach and cheese ravioli with marinara sauce, Caesar salad (no anchovies), watermelon, milk	veggie burger on wholegrain bun with lettuce, cheese, tomato and onion, roasted red potatoes, fruit kebab, milk	aubergine, parmesan, asparagus, wholewheat dinner roll, apricots, milk
cottage cheese with fresh fruit	small quesadilla (vegetarian refried beans, light cheese and wholewheat tortilla)	wholegrain bagel with light veggie cream cheese

Resources

www.vrg.org

www.nal.usda.gov/fnic/etext/000058.html

www.vegetariannutrition.net

www.vegsoc.org/health

Messina, V., Messina, M. *The Vegetarian Way* (1996, Three Rivers Press)

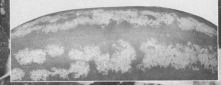

Note: Where "milk" is listed on the menu, it may be cow's milk, fortified soya milk or fortified rice milk. If soya or rice milk, it should be fortified with calcium and vitamin D. When buying juice, buy a version fortified with calcium.

LACTOSE-RESTRICTED DIET

LONG-TERM PLAN

FLEXIBILITY

FAMILY FRIENDLY

COST
●

STRENGTH OF SCIENCE

This plan provides guidelines for those who are lactose intolerant or have difficulty digesting lactose. Those who are allergic to milk will require different dietary precautions.

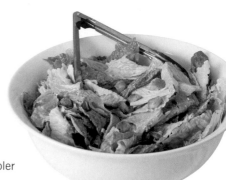

Diet history
Three paediatricians described lactose intolerance in 1901. Earlier diet prescriptions were more restrictive than those currently being followed. These days the level of intolerance (maldigestion) determines the degree of restriction and the dietary strategies required.

How does it work?
During digestion, lactose is broken down into two simpler sugars – glucose and galactose – with the help of the enzyme lactase found in the small intestine. The body's inability to produce any or sufficient quantities of lactase means that milk sugar reaches the colon and cannot be broken down. This causes uncomfortable symptoms such as gas, bloating and/or diarrhoea.

Although there are a variety of strategies, they all basically do one or both of the following: decrease the amount of lactose consumed or break milk sugar down into glucose and galactose before it is ingested. Milk is avoided to decrease the amount of lactose that is consumed and that includes evaporated milk, ice cream, cream and products

sample menu

Include lactose-free or low-lactose milk, aged

	saturday	sunday	monday	tuesday
morning	wheat flakes cereal, lactose-free low-fat milk, oatmeal bagel, margarine, banana	peanut butter, banana smoothie with ½ glass skimmed milk*, wholewheat crackers	porridge with lactose-free low-fat milk, wholewheat toast, grapefruit sections, coffee	omelette with mixed vegetables, toast, coffee with lactose-free low-fat milk
lunch	Caesar salad with grilled chicken and low-calorie dressing, multigrain roll, water	French onion soup, ½ tuna sandwich with lettuce and tomatoes, lemonade	greens with ham and cheddar cheese cubes, Italian dressing, diet cola	vegetable, bean and pasta soup, Caesar salad, wholegrain roll, orange-pineapple juice blend
supper	grilled tilapia, broccoli with cheese, red potatoes, roll, orange juice	cos lettuce salad with grilled chicken strips and Italian dressing, multigrain bread, sparkling water	minced turkey and bean chilli in tomato sauce, brown rice, steamed green beans, fresh limeade	wholewheat pizza with veggies, grapefruit, iced tea
snack 1	lactose-free milk vanilla pudding	fruit ice	orange juice spritzer, wholewheat crackers	crackers, hot chocolate with lactose-free milk
snack 2	popcorn, cranberry juice	pear with vanilla yogurt topping	bagel, margarine, apple juice	tropical fruit salad, rye breadsticks

containing milk or milk powder. Lactose-free or low-lactose versions of the product – such as low-lactose or lactose-free milk – can be used instead. Mature cheeses and yogurts may be consumed if the milk has been fermented and no additional milk added.

Lactase can be purchased over the counter in pill form and taken prior to consumption to break down sugar into glucose and galactose before it is ingested. A total avoidance of unfermented dairy products is not needed generally and the dieter can try any of the following strategies: drinking small amounts of milk with other foods; focusing on mature cheeses; introducing dairy foods then slowly and gradually increasing the amount; using lactose-free milk and milk products; consuming bio-active yogurt.

Pros and cons

This plan will help someone with true intolerance to enjoy dairy products without experiencing any discomfort.

When following this lactose-intolerance plan, care must be taken to consume the adequate amount of calcium. Anyone who self-diagnoses and wrongly follows this plan may, in fact, have a milk protein allergy.

Is it for you?

This plan will suit anyone who has been medically tested and diagnosed lactose intolerant. Those individuals with a milk allergy should not follow the diet and should seek appropriate counselling for that condition instead.

Availability

All foods in this diet are widely available and can be purchased from any general food shop or supermarket.

Lifestyle changes

None.

What is lactose?

Lactose is the naturally occurring sugar in milk. During digestion, it is broken down into two other sugars, glucose and galactose, with the help of an enzyme called lactase. If you do not produce any or enough lactase, milk sugar cannot be broken down and some physical discomforts occur.

healthy tips

- If you think you are lactose intolerant or have difficulty digesting lactose, do not self-diagnose. Check with your doctor who can look at your medical history, complete a physical examination and conduct a hydrogen breath-test or lactose tolerance test.

cheeses, and bio-active yogurt to increase calcium intake.

wednesday	thursday	friday
wholegrain dry cereal with lactose-free low-fat milk, orange sections, hot tea	cream of wheat with lactose-free low-fat milk, wholewheat toast, pineapple juice	wholewheat bagel with low-fat sausage, coffee with lactose-free low-fat milk
chicken salad sandwich, side salad with vinegar and rapeseed oil dressing, small probiotic yogurt drink	veggie burger and tomato slices on wholewheat bread, fruit salad, iced tea	grilled turkey breast, rice pilaf, steamed carrots, lactose-free milk with chocolate flavouring
fish stewed with onions and tomatoes, yellow rice, Brussels sprouts, sparkling water	herbed lamb chop, mashed cauliflower, sautéed spinach, wholewheat roll, iced tea	veal parmesan with mixed vegetables, side salad, garlic bread, red wine
grape juice, berries on angel cake	tomato juice, rice crackers	berry smoothie
salsa, baked pitta chips, diet soda	baked apple, lactose-free milk	trail mix, orange juice

Resources

www.nationaldairycouncil.org

www.nationaldairycouncil.com

digestive.niddk.nih.gov/ddiseases/pubs/lactoseintolerance

Note: More restrictive plans may not allow any dairy products.
*If tolerated; otherwise use lactose-free or low-lactose milk.

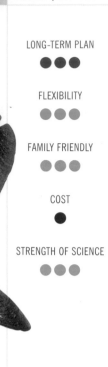

LONG-TERM PLAN
●●●

FLEXIBILITY
●●●

FAMILY FRIENDLY
●●●

COST
●

STRENGTH OF SCIENCE
●●●

LATIN AMERICAN DIET PYRAMID

This healthy food plan incorporates exotic foods from various Latin American cultures to promote healthy eating and fitness.

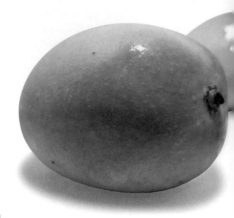

Diet history
The Latin American Diet Pyramid was the third food guide developed by the Oldways Preservation Trust in the 1990s. Its co-founder, environmental activist and Harvard graduate K. Dun Gifford, promoted healthy eating habits based on a philosophy which encouraged demand for traditional foods, sustainable forms of agriculture and an appreciation of global culinary arts. Variations of this diet have traditionally existed in different parts of Latin America where local staples include maize, potatoes, peanuts and dry beans.

A summit held in Mexico City in 2005 further increased international recognition and support for this diet with a consortium of scientific and culinary advisors, industry members, and other specialists advocating healthy living education initiatives focused on its food selection and choice of physical activity.

healthy tips
• Delight your tastebuds with the exotic flavours of the exciting variety of fruits, vegetables and grains included in this eating plan.

How does it work?
The pyramid combines the nutritional merits of traditional indigenous Latin American dishes from the Aztec, Inca and Maya cultures with foods or recipes introduced by the arrival of Columbus and other European explorers.

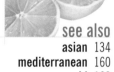

sample menu
The focus is on healthy traditional

	saturday	sunday	monday	tuesday
morning	wholewheat cereal, milk, tomato juice, coffee with milk	baked arepa (cornmeal griddle cake) with cheese, coffee with milk	mango juice, egg-white omelette with peppers, corn tortillas, coffee with milk	wholewheat cereal, milk, banana, coffee with milk
snack	hot chocolate with milk, wholewheat crackers with guava jam	melon salad, iced tea	tropical fruit cup	papaya milkshake, wholewheat toast
lunch	ham and cheese sandwich, orange juice, peanuts	guacamole, mashed beans, wholewheat tortillas, salad	chicken noodle soup, salad with pecans, orange slices	quesadillas, tomato and pepper salad, orange juice
snack	citrus fruit cup with almonds, iced tea	apple, white cheese, wholewheat crackers	white cheese, wholewheat roll, hot chocolate with milk	peanuts, iced tea
dinner	grilled prawns, boiled yucca, carrots, wholewheat rolls	pork loin with chillies, succotash, baked sweet potato	grilled fish, kale, wholewheat tortillas, mixed salad, iced tea	baked pork chop, baked potato, roasted aubergine, wholewheat rolls, hot chocolate with milk

The base of the three-tiered pyramid recommends daily physical activities such as walking and dancing. The first level includes foods from the fruits, vegetables and whole grains, tubers, pasta, beans and nuts categories at every meal. The next level advises eating some fish or shellfish, plant oils or dairy and poultry on a daily basis. The top tier advocates the consumption of meat, sweets and eggs once a week.

The dieter must drink at least six glasses of water a day, with any alcohol consumed in moderation. Some of the menu suggestions include foodstuffs native to the Americas such as amaranth, cacao, chilies, corn, tomato, peanut, potato, quinoa and turkey but also ingredients introduced to the region after colonization by the Spanish. These ingredients include beef, aubergine, kiwi fruit, olives, oranges, soya and courgettes.

Pros and cons

The plan contains useful advice on how to integrate culturally popular foods into a healthy eating pattern supported by scientific research, ecological awareness and regional foods. Unfortunately, the food pyramid does not indicate serving amounts. If the dieter requires a menu with daily portion or food group allocations, other sources have to be consulted.

Is it for you?

It is most likely to appeal to people who enjoy tropical fruit and vegetables, like or are curious about exotic food and culture, or have an adventurous palate.

Availability

Most of the foods in this diet can be purchased from most supermarkets. Look for some of the less well-known ingredients in the ethnic or gourmet aisles. Some fruits or vegetables may be difficult to find or expensive when not in season.

Lifestyle changes

Regular physical activity is recommended.

treats

PICK FROM:

- papaya
- mango
- pineapple
- peanuts
- lime
- guava
- custard apple
- cocoa
- puddings
- biscuits (occasionally)

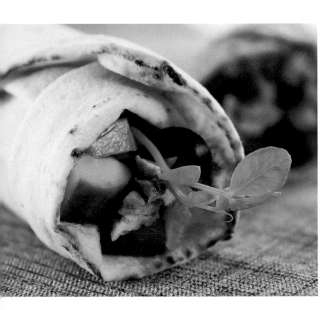

foods such as legumes, squash, seeds, nuts and peppers.

	wednesday	thursday	friday
	orange, porridge with milk, coffee with milk	scrambled eggs, wholewheat toasts, pineapple juice, coffee with milk	porridge with milk, grapefruit, coffee with milk
	tomato juice	apple, iced tea	corn tortilla with cheese
	bean burritos, cactus salad, mixed greens with almonds, pineapple juice	grilled fish, baked ripe plantain, chickpea and quinoa salad, wholewheat roll	vegetable and noodle soup, Caesar salad, wholewheat toasts
	hot chocolate with milk, wholewheat crackers with jam	melon salad, tea	banana, pumpkin seeds
	grilled salmon, wholewheat rolls, courgette/onion sauté iced tea	pasta with tomatoes and cheese, green salad	turkey breast, yellow rice, spinach salad with orange

Note: Where "milk" is mentioned, use low fat to 1% or 2%.

Resources

www.latinonutrition.org/LatinPyramid.html

www.oldwayspt.org

Rodriguez, J. *Contemporary Nutrition for Latinos* (2004, iUniverse)

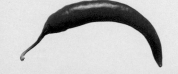

LOW-SODIUM DIET

A low-in-sodium (a table salt component and a natural ingredient) diet prevents or manages certain kinds of diseases and medical conditions.

LONG-TERM PLAN

FLEXIBILITY

FAMILY FRIENDLY

COST

STRENGTH OF SCIENCE

Diet history
The Low-Sodium Diet has been used for many years for patients with high blood pressure, kidney problems, congestive heart failure and water retention (oedema). Very well known and originally used by healthcare practitioners to educate patients, the programme has gained recent popularity among the general public who want to protect their health.

How does it work?
Necessary for maintaining good health, sodium is a naturally occurring mineral found in all kinds of foods. Too much sodium, however, can have detrimental effects. While a healthy adult needs around 500mg daily, the average diet contains around 6,000mg. When present in excess, it can cause thirst, water retention, higher blood pressure and other health conditions.

Some of our sodium intake comes from table salt but the majority stems from the preservatives used in canned and processed foods.

Make sure soups are homemade or purchased with little or no salt added.

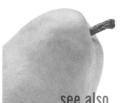

see also
dash 138
tlc 176

sample menu
The Low-Sodium Diet consists of more fresh

	saturday	sunday	monday	tuesday
morning	French toast, grapefruit, skimmed milk	buckwheat pancakes, strawberries, honeydew melon, skimmed milk	breakfast burrito, cantaloupe, skimmed milk	porridge with raisins, orange juice, skimmed milk
lunch	vegetarian chilli, baked potato, low-salt wholewheat crackers, cantaloupe, lemonade	Manhattan-style low-salt clam chowder, low-salt wholewheat crackers, orange, skimmed milk	chicken breast sandwich, baked potato wedges	taco salad with tortilla chips, avocado, skimmed milk
supper	pizza with toppings, green salad, skimmed milk	stir-fried tofu with veggies, brown rice, fruit yogurt, iced tea	grilled salmon, saffron rice with almonds, broccoli, skimmed milk	spinach lasagne with hummus filling, wholewheat dinner roll, skimmed milk
snack 1	wholewheat crackers (no salt)	sunflower seeds (no salt)	orange juice	almonds
snack 2	fruit cocktail in water	banana	carrot sticks	pineapple

weigh this up...

- Instead of adding salt, use low-sodium herbs and spices to enrich your diet. Use allspice or cumin to season meat, or basil and fennel to perk up fish dishes. Onion, oregano and red peppers add pizazz to vegetables. Prepare a combination of herbs and/or spices to create your own seasoning blend.
- Remember to always read the labels on food. Avoid those with the word "sodium" (either alone or in combination with other words) in the ingredients list.

Following the Low-Sodium Diet guidelines means reading food labels and ingredient lists carefully to make healthier and informed choices. Limit the amount of table salt in the preparation of recipes and at mealtimes by opting for salt-free herbs and spices that add variety and flavour.

Pros and cons

This eating strategy avoids the use of table salt and processed or tinned foods that are high in sodium and salt while encouraging the consumption of a variety of fresh foods, herbs and spices. An understanding of the recommendations to follow allows flexible food choices.

The drawback of this diet is its lack of meal plans or caloric recommendations for reducing high-sodium foods.

Is it for you?

A low-sodium diet allows you to consume all kinds of foods, whether high or low in salt, in moderation, and fresh fruit and vegetables are also recommended. Suitable individuals with high blood pressure, kidney disease, oedema and cardiovascular diseases; those at risk of high blood pressure with a family history of heart disease may also benefit. A low-sodium diet limits the amount to the recommended daily dose but without reducing the intake of other vital nutrients, so there is no need for most people to avoid this plan.

Availability

The diet's recommended foods – including fresh or most frozen fruit and vegetables, fresh meat and whole grains prepared without any added salt – are widely available from general food shops nationwide.

Lifestyle changes

Physical activity for 30–45 minutes, three to five times a week, is recommended.

forbidden foods

- pickles
- olives
- cured meats
- canned products (vegetables, soups and meat dishes)
- frozen dinners
- crisps
- crackers
- some cheeses
- cooking wine
- sauerkraut

foods and fewer processed foods.

wednesday	thursday	friday
bran flakes cereal, skimmed milk, banana, wholewheat toast, margarine, prune juice	hard-boiled egg, wholewheat muffin, margarine, jam, grapefruit	puffed wheat cereal, raisins, skimmed milk, banana, wholewheat toast, margarine, jam
tuna sandwich, pear, skimmed milk	minestrone soup with beans, baby carrots, French bread, skimmed milk	smoked turkey sandwich, apple, no-salt-added tomato juice
roast chicken breast, sweet potato, peas and onions, green salad with cider vinegar	rigatoni with meat sauce, spinach salad with tangerine vinaigrette dressing, skimmed milk	grilled T-bone, mashed potatoes, carrots, wholewheat dinner roll, skimmed milk
dried apricots	fruit, yogurt	yogurt
yogurt	apple	raisins

Resources

www.mayoclinic.com/health/food-and-nutrition/AN00350

www.healthsystem.virginia.edu/internet/digestive-health/nutrition/lowsoddiet.cfm

www.nlm.nih.gov/medlineplus/ency/article/002415.htm

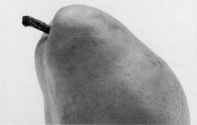

LONG-TERM PLAN

FLEXIBILITY

FAMILY FRIENDLY

COST

●

STRENGTH OF SCIENCE

●

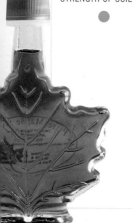

THE MASTER CLEANSER

The Master Cleanser diet is designed to eliminate toxins and cleanse the kidneys and digestive system.

Diet history

Originally popularized by Stanley Burroughs in the 1940s and first published by him in 1976, The Master Cleanser is based on the Lemonade Diet. It is recommended for "all acute and chronic conditions", "when overweight is a problem", "when the digestive system needs a rest", or "when building of body tissue is needed". Two other versions have been published since, both of which refer to the Lemonade Diet. Celebrities have popularized the diet, publicizing its use primarily for cleansing and/or quick weight loss.

How it works

The diet is recommended to be followed for a minimum of ten days, up to a maximum of forty, and is purported to meet all dietary requirements during this time. The lemon drink taken six to twelve times a day during the waking period comprises the diet. No other food should be taken during the full period of this diet. Supplements are not permitted. Extra water may be taken as desired. A laxative herb tea from a health food shop may be used to increase elimination each night and first thing in the morning.

The rationale for the recipe that makes up the lemon drink is presumed to be associated with the unique characteristics of each ingredient. Lemons or limes must be fresh – and organic is

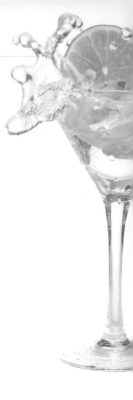

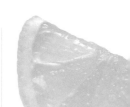

sample menu

Consume the diet's lemon drink* 6–12 times a

	saturday	sunday	monday	tuesday
breakfast	lemon drink*	lemon drink*	lemon drink*	lemon drink*
lunch	lemon drink*	lemon drink*	lemon drink*	lemon drink*
dinner	lemon drink*	lemon drink*	lemon drink*	lemon drink*
snack 1 (3–9 times per day)	lemon drink*	lemon drink*	lemon drink*	lemon drink*

recommended – and blending a part of the lemon skin and pulp with the lemon juice results in further cleansing and provides a laxative effect. The maple syrup (darker grades, B and C are preferred) is described as containing a large variety of vitamins and minerals. Honey is not to be substituted for the maple sugar and should never be ingested internally at any time. Cayenne pepper adds B and C vitamins, which the diet claims is needed to break up mucus, and "increase warmth by building the blood for an additional lift".

The first and second day following the diet, add several 230ml glasses of fresh orange juice and extra water as desired. On the third day, add orange juice in the morning, raw fruit for lunch and fruit or raw vegetable salad at night. The recommended diet for life is a natural vegetarian diet.

Pros and cons

On a short-term basis, the diet may not cause harm. However, the adequacy of nutrient intake is questionable: each drink contains approximately 115 calories with virtually no fat, 0.4 grams of protein and 29 grams of carbohydrate. For people who have certain diseases, especially kidney failure or cancer, this diet could promote further illness or malnutrition.

The current scientific data does not support that fasting, extremely low calorie intake, nor lemons cleanse or rid the body of toxins, and although the diet may not be harmful for just a few days, with long-term use it can slow down metabolism, cause muscle wasting and be harmful to some body organs.

Is it for you?

This plan would suit those who want a radical change from their usual diets, have health issues that they feel will benefit, or are interested in attempting to cleanse the system. The diet should be avoided by persons with diabetes, kidney disease, cancer, irritable bowel syndrome or other illnesses. A person interested in trying this diet should first consult a doctor.

Availability

The recommended ingredients are widely available in grocery stores.

Lifestyle changes

None, other than the diet.

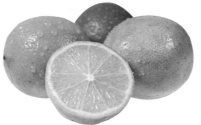
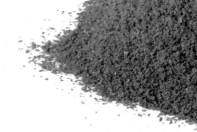

day for at least 10 days.

wednesday	thursday	friday
lemon drink*	lemon drink*	lemon drink*
lemon drink*	lemon drink*	lemon drink*
lemon drink*	lemon drink*	lemon drink*
lemon drink*	lemon drink*	lemon drink*

* Recipe in Burroughs, S. *The Master Cleanser – with special needs and problems*.

Resources

www.mastercleanser.com

www.webmd.com/food-recipes/features/detox-diets-purging-myths

Burroughs, S. *The Master Cleanser – with special needs and problems* (1976, Burroughs Books) Revised Edition 1993, Burroughs, A.

Glickman, P. *Lose Weight, Have More Energy & Be Happier in 10 Days* (2005, Peter Glickman)

Woloshyn, T. *Complete Master Cleanse: A Step by Step Guide to Maximizing the Benefits of the Lemonade Diet* (2007, Ulysses Press)

MEDITERRANEAN FOOD PYRAMID

A lifestyle eating guide based on the dietary patterns of Italy, Greece, parts of North Africa and the Middle East.

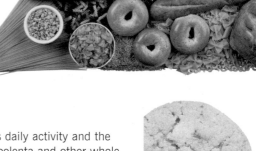

LONG-TERM PLAN

FLEXIBILITY

FAMILY FRIENDLY

COST

STRENGTH OF SCIENCE

Diet history

Borrowing heavily from the cultural food patterns of over 15 countries based around the Mediterranean region, this diet plan was originally developed by the Oldways Preservation Trust, an organization concerned with promoting healthy eating based on traditional food patterns, sustainable agricultural practices and an appreciation for culturally influenced cuisine. These principles have produced several diet books and many associations have incorporated or developed variations of the original food pyramid model.

How does it work?

The Mediterranean Food Pyramid recommends daily activity and the following foods: bread, rice, pasta, couscous, polenta and other whole grains, potatoes, fruits, beans, legumes, nuts, vegetables, olive oil,

see also
asian 134
latin american 154
mypyramid 162

sample menu

Emphasize daily foods from plant sources and

	saturday	sunday	monday	tuesday
morning	poached egg, pitta bread, ½ grapefruit, tea, water	polenta, cheese wedge, grapes, coffee	porridge, orange slices, coffee	yogurt, fresh fruit, multigrain bread, coffee, water
lunch	potato wedges, sardines in tomato, onion and olive oil, Greek salad	flat bread, lentil soup, curried cauliflower, pear-walnut salad	onion baked potatoes, chicken breast, spinach salad with olives, water	rice with pistachios and broad beans, tossed green salad, olive oil, figs
supper	vine leaves, white beans and avocado salad, tabbouleh, wine	pasta primavera with chicken strips, sliced cucumbers and tomatoes with olive oil, water	vegetable soup, pasta with pesto, avocado and watercress salad	grilled fish, couscous with raisins, herbed broccoli, flat bread
snack 1	cheese, olives	nectarines	yogurt, sliced berries	grapes
snack 2	pistachios	grapes	olives	fruit ice

cheese and yogurt. Fish, poultry, eggs and sweets are limited to weekly consumption, and meat reduced to just once a month.

The pyramid's composition is based on the culinary heritage of countries where the dietary emphasis is on locally grown and minimally processed foods, a high consumption of fresh fruit and vegetables, bread and other cereals (especially whole grains), potatoes, beans, nuts, seeds and olive oil. Moderate amounts of dairy, including yogurt, cheese, fish, poultry and eggs, can be consumed, with red meat a rare treat. Wine may be enjoyed in low to moderate amounts during meals.

In recent years the plan's profile has been raised further by the link found between the reduced risk of heart disease and the presence of olive oil and reduced saturated fats in diet. More studies, however, are needed to discover which specific dietary components, or their combination with other lifestyle factors, most impact on heart disease rates.

Pros and cons
Based both on scientific and cultural findings, and a philosophy of supporting traditional food habits and leading an active lifestyle, the Mediterranean Food Pyramid Diet incorporates healthy foods from regions with cuisines that are popular worldwide.

The pyramid, however, does not indicate serving sizes or amounts, and the frequency of consumption for certain kinds of food may vary by country. The presence of olive oil is encouraged but caution must be taken to avoid eating too much of any type of fat.

Is it for you?
This plan will appeal to people who enjoy the freshness of Mediterranean ingredients and like having lots of fruit and vegetables, beans and nuts.

Availability
Most of the ingredients in this diet can be bought from any general food shop. The fresh fruit and vegetables, whole grains and low-fat dairy sections in a supermarket will stock many of the foods.

Lifestyle changes
Daily physical activity is integral to the plan.

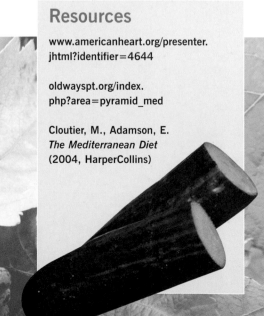

treats
- olives
- grapes
- nuts
- pastries and biscuits (occasionally)

healthy tips
- Use puréed white beans, chickpeas, lentils, aubergine, tomatoes, garlic, capers and olive oil to prepare delicious dips for snacks. Serve with wholewheat pitta bread or raw vegetable sticks.

moderate amounts of cheese, yogurt and olive oil.

wednesday	thursday	friday
omelette with spinach and feta cheese, flatbread, tea	wholewheat bread, mascarpone cheese, marmalade, coffee, water	porridge with strawberries, Italian bread, coffee
pasta and white bean salad, tomato slices with mozzarella cheese, water	chicken soup, roll, large salad with greens, feta cheese, chickpeas, olive oil and lemon	cheese polenta, chicken sautéed in olive oil, steamed artichokes, pickled beetroot
olive bread, grilled prawns, basil, cucumber and tomato salad, orzo with pine nuts, wine	lemon chicken soup, cod, baked red potatoes, roasted mushrooms and aubergine	stewed calamari risotto with peppers and mushrooms, tossed green salad, water
almonds	figs	orange
cheese and fruit	olives	date and nut cookie

Resources
www.americanheart.org/presenter.jhtml?identifier=4644

oldwayspt.org/index.php?area=pyramid_med

Cloutier, M., Adamson, E. *The Mediterranean Diet* (2004, HarperCollins)

LONG-TERM PLAN

FLEXIBILITY

FAMILY FRIENDLY

COST

STRENGTH OF SCIENCE

MYPYRAMID PLAN

This personalized eating model is based on the various food groups and divided up by calorie levels to help you find the one right for you.

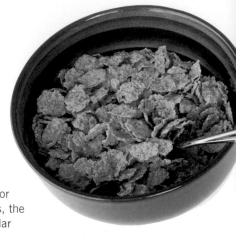

Diet history

This dietary plan is the United States government's current food model. The US Department of Agriculture (USDA) first published general dietary recommendations in 1894 followed by a food guide for young children in 1916. First published in the 1940s, the wheel-shaped food guide was replaced by a rectangular equivalent from the 1950s through to the 1970s.

The recently published MyPyramid model is well known but some may be more familiar with the previous Food Guide Pyramid and not realize that this is its replacement. The 1992 Food Guide Pyramid was most recently updated in 2005.

These amendments were necessary as they reflect a progression in the new scientific findings for promoting overall health and provide the general public with a practical, up-to-date, flexible approach to healthy eating. There are supporters and critics of MyPyramid, which has resulted in the development of alternative plans by some groups and organizations.

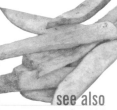

see also
asian 134
latin american 154
mediterranean 160

sample menu

Menu available at www.mypyramid.gov

	saturday	sunday	monday	tuesday	
morning	French toast with maple syrup, ½ grapefruit, fat-free milk	buckwheat pancakes with maple syrup, strawberries, honeydew melon, fat-free milk	breakfast burrito on flour tortilla with black beans and salsa, orange juice	porridge with raisins, fat-free milk, orange juice	
lunch	vegetarian chilli, canteloupe, grape spritzer	clam chowder with fat-free milk, wholewheat crackers, lemonade	roast beef sandwich on wholegrain bread with lettuce and tomatoes, potato wedges	taco salad with minced turkey, beans and low-fat cheese	
supper	Hawaiian pizza with thick-cut bacon, onions and mushrooms, green salad, skimmed milk	vegetable stir-fry with tofu, bok choy and peppers, brown rice	grilled stuffed salmon, rice with almonds, steamed broccoli, skimmed milk	spinach lasagne, wholewheat dinner roll, skimmed milk	
snack	wholewheat crackers, hummus, fruit cocktail	sunflower seeds, banana, low-fat fruit yogurt	cantaloupe	almonds, pineapple, raisins	

healthy tips
MyPyramid suggests:
- Eating more fruit, vegetables, whole grains, fat-free or low-fat dairy.
- Making half of the grains eaten of the whole grain variety.
- Eating less foods that are high in saturated or trans fats, added sugars, cholesterol, salt and alcohol.

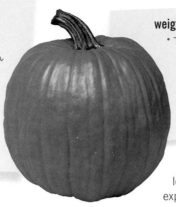

weigh this up...
- The "discretionary calorie allowance" is the amount of calories left over from food intake after the calories from all the food groups have been accounted for.

How does it work?
The following principles underpin the rationale for MyPyramid: that one size does not fit all; that daily physical activity is essential; that goals should be based on gradual not sudden improvement; finally, that eating should be based on moderation, proportionality (how much to have from each group) and variety (eating foods from different categories daily). Its dietary guidelines emphasize the consumption of fruits, vegetables, whole grains, fat-free or low-fat milk and dairy products; lean meats, poultry, fish, beans, eggs and nuts; and a low intake of saturated fats, trans fats, cholesterol, salt (sodium) and added sugars.

The food groups include fruit, vegetables, grains, meat and beans, milk and oils. MyPyramid uses "discretionary calories" and advises on the amounts required from each food group based on nutrient intakes at 12 different energy levels, ranging from 1,000 to 3,200 calories, at 200-calorie increments.

Pros and cons
This flexible plan provides options based on caloric content and informs you on the amounts from each food group that are needed by an individual based on his or her activity levels. The illustrated food guide, however, is not self-explanatory and users must access the website to obtain any tailormade information.

Is it for you?
The programme is designed for healthy individuals who want generic guidelines about what and how much to eat from the various food groups as assessed by food intake and physical activity. People with special needs or medical conditions should consult a doctor or a registered dietician.

Availability
Any of the recommended foods in this diet can be bought from any general food shop or supermarket.

Lifestyle changes
Daily physical activity is recommended as part of the MyPyramid Plan.

wednesday	thursday	friday
bran flakes cereal with fat-free milk, banana, wholewheat toast, margarine, prune juice	medium grapefruit, hard-boiled egg, wholewheat muffin, margarine, jam	cold cereal with raisins, fat-free milk, banana, wholewheat toast, margarine, jam
tuna sandwich on rye bread with lettuce and tomato, pear, fat-free milk	white bean vegetable soup, breadsticks, carrot sticks, fat-free milk	smoked turkey sandwich with lettuce and tomato, apple, tomato juice
roast chicken breast, baked sweet potatoes, peas and onions, wholewheat roll, green salad	rigatoni with meat sauce, spinach salad with walnuts and tangerines, skimmed milk	boiled top-loin steak, mashed potatoes, steamed carrots, wholewheat dinner roll, skimmed milk
dried apricots, low-fat fruit yogurt	low-fat fruit yogurt	low-fat fruit yogurt

Resources
www.mypyramid.gov

www.mypyramid.gov/professionals/food_tracking_wksht.html

health.learninginfo.org/food-pyramid.htm

LONG-TERM PLAN
● ● ●

FLEXIBILITY
● ●

FAMILY FRIENDLY
● ● ●

COST
●

STRENGTH OF SCIENCE
● ●

OMEGA PLAN

This Mediterranean-style diet advocates the moderate consumption of healthy fats to make up 30–35 per cent of the total number of calories allowed.

Diet history
Although this particular plan was first published by Artemis P. Simopoulos, MD, and Jo Robinson in 1998, a diet with a moderate intake of "healthy" fats is found in various other diets and food guides.

How does it work?
According to the Omega diet, the "missing link" which made the health and longevity of the people of Crete superior to those from other communities were foods higher in Omega-3 fatty acids and the ratio of Omega-6 to Omega-3 fatty acids.

   According to the diet, there are "bad" and "good" fats. To decrease the risk of coronary heart disease, diabetes and obesity, "good" fats (unsaturated fats) should be eaten in the correct ratios and in moderate amounts with "bad" fats (saturated and trans fats) cut out of the diet. Saturated fats are found in meat, dairy and tropical oils such as palm and coconut oils. Trans fats, the by-product of the hydrogenation of oils (the process of adding a hydrogen molecule to

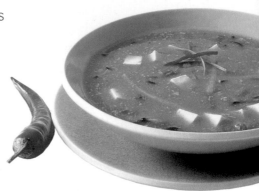

Hot and sour soup that contains tofu willl be a good source of Omega-3 fatty acids.

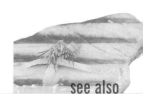

see also
mediterranean 160
perricone 168

sample menu

Include generous amounts of fruits, vegetables,

	saturday	sunday	monday	tuesday
morning	orange sections, buckwheat pancakes, with flaxseed, maple syrup	bagel, smoked salmon, tomato slices, red onions, orange juice	cantaloupe, plain bagel, tomato slices, 30g mozzarella cheese	honeydew, wholegrain toast, rapeseed butter, poached egg
lunch	tomato juice, pasta primavera with walnut pesto, honey flax bread	bean soup, strawberry, nut and spinach salad, honey and olive oil dressing, pitta bread	chicken salad with olive oil mayonnaise, green salad, flat multigrain bread	vegetable soup, green salad with walnut oil dressing and flaxseed, wholewheat pitta
supper	pot roast, baked potato, steamed carrots, wholewheat roll, rapeseed butter	grilled tuna steak, bulgur with mushrooms, sautéed kale with olive oil, grilled tomatoes	baked salmon, edamame beans, purslane and mesclun salad with olive oil dressing, wholewheat roll	grilled chicken breast, acorn squash with rapeseed butter, peas and carrots
snack 1	figs in light syrup	grapes	pear and low-fat cottage cheese	orange walnut salad
snack 2	walnuts	olives, baked pitta chips	hummus, courgette sticks	skimmed milk hot chocolate

make a liquid oil solid), are even worse and have been associated with certain kinds of cancers.

"Good" fats such as olive and rapeseed oils or oils with essential fatty acids are strongly encouraged as they are necessary for growth and development. Omega-6 fatty acids are mostly found in vegetable oils (corn, safflower and sunflower). Omega-3 fatty acids are found in fish and seafood, rapeseed oil and green leafy vegetables.

The scientific data supports the notion that moderate amounts of Omega-3 and Omega-6 promote good health, especially cardiovascular. The book, however, purports that the Omega Plan should be used for many other conditions for which the current available data is preliminary and/or inconclusive.

The Omega Plan promotes eating a variety of healthy foods, including seven or more servings of fruit and vegetables, vegetable proteins (such as beans) and a reduction of trans and saturated fats.

Pros and cons

The guide provides options for those who want to follow the diet solely for weight loss and offers tips on grocery shopping and setting up an "Omega kitchen" at home. Although eating Omega-3 rich foods is highly recommended, the dieter is given the choice of taking

treats

PICK FROM:
- 100-calorie healthy snacks that include 30g cheese, 150g fresh apricots, ½ glass 1% chocolate milk
- 110g crab meat
- 1 frozen fruit bar or 12 large olives

supplements instead. These pills, however, cannot counteract the effects of poor diet.

Is it for you?

The Omega Plan will appeal to individuals looking for a programme that is moderate in fat but includes health-promoting fats and fights the risk of developing some chronic diseases. Anyone with a medical condition, such as diabetes, should consult a doctor or a registered dietician to determine whether they should and if possible how best to follow this type of diet.

Availability

Most of these foods are widely available from general food shops and supermarkets.

Lifestyle changes

Keep a food, mood and exercise diary to identify and fight eating triggers.

healthy tips

- Stock up on Omega-3 and Omega-6 fatty acids found in these oils: rapeseed, olive, flaxseed, safflower, sunflower; and also in rapeseed- or olive-oil-based mayonnaise.

legumes, fatty fish, walnuts, flaxseed and greens.

wednesday	thursday	friday
grapefruit sections, muesli with flaxseed, skimmed milk	wholewheat muffin, low-fat cottage cheese, jam	mixed berries, egg-white omelette with spinach, wholewheat toast, jam
vegetable broth, Greek salad with olive oil dressing, pitta bread, canola butter	turkey sandwich, tomato and cucumber slices with olive oil	hot-sour soup, veggie burger with rapeseed mayonnaise, sautéed vegetables
grilled lamb chop, mashed cauliflower, Brussels sprouts, wholewheat roll	miso soup, pork loin stir-fry, brown rice, rocket with ginger and rapeseed oil	grilled trout, butter beans and corn (succotash) with rapeseed butter, green salad with olive oil dressing
mixed berry salad	strawberries	frozen fruit bar
grape juice	banana	30g low-fat cheese

Resources

www.oznet.kstate.edu/humannutrition/omega1.htm

www.dietwords.com/theomega_diet.shtml

Simopoulos, A.P., Robinson, J. *The Omega Plan* (1998, HarperCollins)

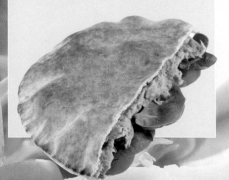

LONG-TERM PLAN

FLEXIBILITY

FAMILY FRIENDLY

COST

STRENGTH OF SCIENCE

OVEREATERS ANONYMOUS (OA)

This no-diet programme provides social and spiritual support to achieve abstinence from compulsive overeating.

Diet history

Based on a modified version of the first Twelve-Step Programme of Alcoholics Anonymous, Overeaters Anonymous was founded in 1960 by two individuals struggling with compulsive eating who wanted to find a new way to overcome their obsession with food. Today there are around 70,000 members and OA meetings take place in about 60 different countries worldwide.

How does it work?

Although OA does not prescribe or endorse any form of eating, it recommends that each individual seek out nutritional advice from a doctor or qualified dietician and determine a well-balanced personal plan that will promote physical recovery from the disorder known as compulsive overeating.

Emotional and spiritual recovery is built in as a component of the program and is accomplished via a number of strategies and techniques. Sponsorship by other OA members is an integral tool and suggested as a means to recovery. This includes being available on a one-to-one support basis and assisting with understanding how the programme works but only when the other person expresses a desire to do so and is ready. Sponsors have followed the recommended steps of the programme themselves and are willing to help new recruits complete their Twelve Steps by participating in the Twelve Traditions of the programme.

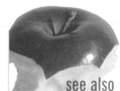

see also
intuitive eating 148

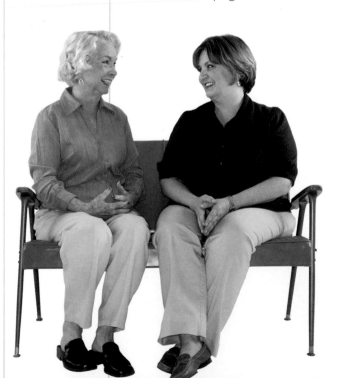

weigh this up...
Consider the following:
- Does your eating behaviour make you or others unhappy?
- Do you eat to escape from your worries or troubles?
- Are you comfortable discussing feelings in a group setting?

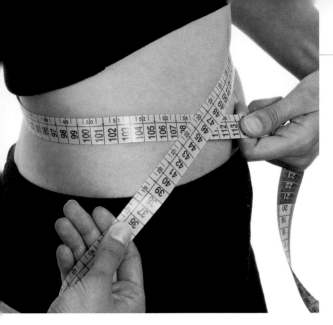

The defining tool of OA is the free meetings that can be attended throughout the world. OA is self-supporting and depends solely on the contributions of its dedicated membership; however, individuals may attend meetings without making a contribution. The purpose of these get-togethers is to furnish a forum for members to share their "experience, strength and hope" to advance and maintain their recovery from food obsession.

OA is not affiliated to any public or private organization, nor is it associated with any religious group. Additional features include sharing one-to-one with other members by means of frequent telephone calls, keeping a diary of thoughts and feelings, reading OA-approved pamphlets and books, and the philosophy of anonymity and service. As a key principle of OA anonymity ensures its members are not exploited or that their own personal sharing and membership are not publicly divulged. Service refers to the OA philosophy of "carrying the message to the compulsive overeater who still suffers", which includes any act that helps to continue the programme. This ensures that the opportunities of OA will be available to all who may desire it in the future.

The Overeaters Anonymous Organization publishes many pamphlets and books to assist members in following the programme. The cost is minimal or free of charge to persons who are not able to afford it. While not necessarily recommending a specific food plan, the OA does distribute literature to help members begin to change their eating behaviours. *A Plan of Eating: A Tool for Living: One Day at a Time* is one such pamphlet that covers important elements for abstinence from compulsive overeating, including using a personal eating plan, and identifying high-risk situations. Consistent with the OA philosophy, however, the pamphlet does not provide any specific food plans.

Pros and cons

The programme promotes the idea that each person should consult a nutritionist in advance to determine specific needs and plan a well-balanced, tailored food plan. The emphasis on healthy eating is established by a holistic approach that attends to the physical, spiritual and emotional needs of its members.

This kind of spiritual focus may deter some individuals from embracing the programme's core concepts. A self-examination of feelings, thoughts, motives and high levels of commitment is needed to incorporate OA principles into your daily lifestyle, and this may be more than some individuals need or want.

Is it for you?

Overeaters Anonymous is suitable for individuals wishing to discover a non-diet lifestyle stategy that focuses on the non-food-related issues that may be contributing to overeating problems. This approach will work better for people who are comfortable in group settings where thoughts and feelings can be openly discussed.

People looking for a diet that is food-focused or a strictly behavioural approach to weight loss and who are not comfortable with group therapy should avoid the plan. Anyone who is uncomfortable with a spiritual or "high-power" method may not find the programme suitable.

Availability

Each individual's eating plan will vary according to his or her specific requirements.

Lifestyle changes

OA encompasses a lifestyle-change approach to overcome the power of compulsive eating. This spiritual-based programme is a "fellowship" of individuals who share their problems with overeating and their methods of recovery. OA offers the necessary tools to assist members in changing their lifestyle to achieve and maintain abstinence. They include sponsorship, meetings, telephone, writing, literature, anonymity and service. The programme does not dictate or require any level of commitment; for success, however, it is recommended that individuals attend frequent meetings, follow the Twelve Steps and acquire a sponsor.

Resources

Elisabeth, L. *Twelve Steps for Overeaters*
(1993, Hazelden Publications)

Overeaters Anonymous **(2001, Overeaters Anonymous)**

www.oa.org

THE PERRICONE PROMISE

The Perricone Promise is that if you follow this diet, you will look and feel ten years younger in just 28 days.

LONG-TERM PLAN
●●

FLEXIBILITY
●●

FAMILY FRIENDLY
●

COST
●●

STRENGTH OF SCIENCE
●●

Diet history
Published in 2004, *The Perricone Promise* was written by Nicolas Perricone, MD, a board certified dermatologist who is an adjunct professor at the Michigan State University College of Human Medicine. Dr Perricone is also author of the best-selling *The Wrinkle Cure* and *The Perricone Prescription*.

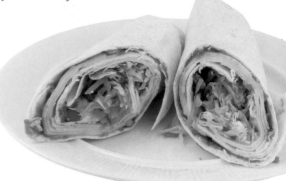

Chicken salad wrap.

How does it work
The programme includes three steps: diet, supplements and topicals. The diet includes "ten superfoods" to reduce inflammation and rejuvenate the skin and body. These are acai berries, allium, barley, young cereal grasses (eg barley or wheat), blue green algae, buckwheat, beans and lentils, hot peppers, nuts and seeds, sprouts and yogurt. In addition, many herbs and spices are recommended.

The recommended supplements include those for anti-glycation, fat metabolizers/energy boosters, anti-ageing/anti-inflammatory, wound healing and wrinkle prevention.

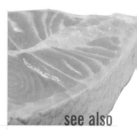

see also
omega 164

sample menu

The plan emphasizes eating superfoods and

	saturday	sunday	monday	tuesday
morning	2 links turkey or tofu sausage, 2 boiled eggs, 200g cooked barley, 240ml green tea/water	80g salmon, 100g barley, ½ tsp cinnamon, 1 tbsp berries, 240ml green tea/water	1 boiled egg, 110g cottage cheese with 1 tbsp ground flaxseed, 25g berries, 240ml green tea/water	omelette: 2 whole eggs and 2 egg whites, 1 slice turkey bacon, 1 kiwi fruit, 240ml green tea/water
lunch	prawn cocktail*, ½ avocado, 1 apple, 240ml water	Caesar salad*, grilled chicken, cantaloupe, 240ml water	Greek salad*, grilled chicken, 1 apple, 240ml water	110g hummus*, 110g grilled salmon, 2 celery sticks, 1 apple, 240ml water
supper	lemon chicken*, oat pilaf*, mixed fruit plate, 240ml water, 2 Norwegian fish oil capsules	savoury halibut*, 100g buckwheat pilaf, 240ml water	stuffed peppers*, green salad, olive oil and lemon juice dressing, 240ml water	curried prawns*, 100g barley, green salad, olive oil and lemon juice dressing, 240ml water
snack 1	1 boiled egg, 1 apple, 3 walnuts, 240ml water	yogurt or kefir smoothie, 240ml water	110g cottage cheese, 1 apple, 240ml water	yogurt or kefir smoothie, 240ml water
snack 2	110g cottage cheese, 1 tbsp pumpkin seeds, 240ml water	1 boiled egg, 1 apple, 3 walnuts, 240ml water	15–30g sliced turkey, 3 olives, 3 strawberries, 240ml water	110g cottage cheese, 1 tbsp ground flaxseed, 35g cherries, 240ml water

The topical treatments recommended to improve the skin's appearance are alpha lipoic acid, thymosin beta 4 and neuropeptides.

This three-pronged approach claims to revitalize skin and hair, strengthen the immune system, promote heart health, decrease the risk of certain cancers, and produce a younger, healthier face and body.

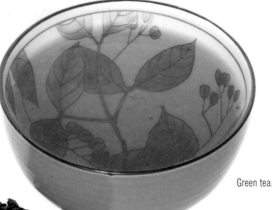

Green tea.

Pros and cons

Many of the recommendations and tips for the 28 days increase the nutrient density of the diet and are positive for that reason.

The supplements, topicals and some of the superfoods may be expensive and their use for "looking younger" and /or "living longer" has not been completely verified by research. To follow the plan every day, the diet, supplements and topics require significant investment of time and money. The Perricone Promise is that after 28 days, readers will look and feel ten years younger, which would be hard to prove or disprove. Presumably, readers would have to follow the plan for the rest of their life to preserve any change seen in the first 28 days.

Is it for you?

This will appeal to persons who like fish, especially salmon, and to those interested in looking young and feeling well as they age. People with gastrointestinal (GI) disorders or allergies who cannot eat nuts, seafood, hot peppers, or other superfoods should avoid the diet.

Availability

Some of the superfoods may be hard to find in some areas as they are primarily sold in speciality or exclusive grocery shops.

Lifestyle changes

Exercise is described as an important factor in regulating neuropeptides. Three types are recommended – weight resistance, cardiovascular or aerobic exercise, and flexibility. Pilates is particularly recommended.

taking supplements to look younger.

wednesday	thursday	friday	
80g salmon, 170g porridge, ½ tsp cinnamon, honeydew, 240ml green tea/water	1 boiled egg, yogurt or kefir smoothie*, 3 macadamia nuts, 240ml green tea/water	omelette: 2 whole eggs and 2 egg whites, 3 almonds, 240ml green tea/water	**Resources**
turkey burger*, green salad, olive oil and lemon juice dressing, 50g berries, 240ml water	chicken salad wrap*, salad or sliced tomatoes, cantaloupe, 240ml water	chicken soup*, 1 pear, 240ml water	www.webmd.com/diet/perricone-diet-what-it-is www.twbookmark.com
80g salmon with lemon, cantaloupe, 240ml water	two-bean turkey/tofu chilli*, green salad, olive oil and lemon juice dressing, 240ml water	lentil or turkey soup*, 80g chicken, green salad, olive oil and lemon juice dressing, 240ml water	Perricone, N. *The Perricone Promise* (2004, Warner Books)
110g hummus*, 2 celery sticks, 3 almonds, 240ml water	30–55g sliced turkey, 3 walnuts, 1 apple, 240ml water	80g plain yogurt, 1 packet pure acai, 1 tbsp sunflower seeds, 240ml water	
1 boiled egg, 3 cherry tomatoes, 3 macadamia nuts, 240ml water	100g cottage cheese, 1 tbsp sunflower seeds, 1 kiwi fruit, 240ml water	30g sliced turkey, 3 olives, 3 cherry tomatoes, 240ml water	

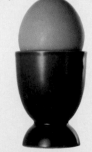

Note: Daily supplements include 2 high-quality Norwegian fish oil capsules, 1 neuropeptide supplement with lunch and 2 high-quality Norwegian fish oil capsules.
*Recipes included in *The Perricone Promise*.

PREGNANCY DIET

This diet recommends adequate amounts of nutrient-dense foods and drinks to promote the health of mother and baby.

LONG-TERM PLAN

FLEXIBILITY

FAMILY FRIENDLY

COST

STRENGTH OF SCIENCE

Diet history
During the 1950s, the ideal weight gain during pregnancy was considered to be 12.5kg (27lb), which included the extra fat stores needed to prepare the mother for breastfeeding. This view held until the 1990s.
Currently, there is no one "number" that is considered the desired gestational weight gain. Instead, recommendations are based on pre-pregnancy body mass index (BMI); however, a weight gain of 11.5–16kg (25–35lb) during pregnancy is considered average and realistic. It is now known that too little weight gain during pregnancy may potentially have a negative health impact on the baby.

How does it work?
Nutrition during pregnancy can affect the unborn child. The goal is for the mother to maintain an adequate nutritional status and, in doing so,

Breakfast, such as this omelette, is an important part of a healthy pregnancy diet.

see also
grazing 116
mediterranean 160
mypyramid 162

sample menu

A well-planned pregnancy diet is also a healthy

	saturday	sunday	monday	tuesday
morning	wholegrain banana and walnut pancakes, lean or soya sausage, nectarine, skimmed milk	scrambled egg, wholewheat bagel, fresh fruit, calcium-fortified orange juice	wholegrain bagel with peanut butter, skimmed milk, banana	porridge, hard-boiled egg, calcium-fortified orange juice, honeydew
lunch	grilled cheese sandwich on wholegrain bread, tomato bisque soup, pear slices, skimmed milk	tuna salad on lettuce with wholegrain crackers, vegetable sticks, fresh pineapple, skimmed milk	turkey sandwich on wholegrain bread, vegetable soup, apple slices, skimmed milk	vegetable pizza, plain yogurt topped with strawberries and muesli, skimmed milk
supper	spinach lasagne, Italian bread, garden salad, fresh fruit, skimmed milk	baked ham, mange-tout, jasmine rice, melon, skimmed milk	salmon, steamed asparagus, brown rice, fresh blueberries, skimmed milk	baked chicken, steamed green beans, baked potato with margarine, cantaloupe, skimmed milk
snack 1	courgette sticks with hummus	low-fat fruit smoothie	crackers	low-fat cottage cheese with fruit
snack 2	fresh fruit	low-fat cottage cheese with fruit	fresh fruit	light popcorn
snack 3	rice cake	fresh fruit	low-fat yogurt	carrot sticks with light ranch dressing

healthy tips

- Avoid marlin, shark, swordfish and similar fish at the top of the food chain.
- Do not eat raw or undercooked fish or shellfish.
- Eat iron-rich foods with foods or drinks high in vitamin C to increase iron absorption.
- Avoid soft cheeses such as feta and brie.
- Eat folate- and calcium-rich foods and drinks.

certain nutrients are highlighted and emphasized. One important nutrient is folate, of which an adequate intake prior to pregnancy and especially during the first few weeks of pregnancy is critical to preventing neural tube defects.

Calcium is also emphasized to build strong bones. Absorption of this mineral actually increases during pregnancy. Extra protein is needed to support the continuous growth of the baby. Additional iron is needed due to the increase in blood volume. Also, consuming excessive, oily fish can be harmful to the baby, as they can contain toxins such as mercury.

Including three nutrient-rich snacks between meals to reduce meal size is important, especially during the third trimester when reflux may become more of a problem.

Pros and cons

The diet is rich in nutrients, such as folate, calcium, iron and protein. It promotes satiety with consumption of three meals and three snacks a day, and healthy food choices, which should be followed postpartum.

Eating throughout the day may become challenging, especially if feeling nauseous. If portion sizes are too big, excessive calories may be consumed, which can cause excessive weight gain.

Is it for you?

This plan is designed for the pregnant woman; it is healthy and also appropriate for most individuals.

Availability

The foods in this diet are all easily accessible and available. There are no special-order foods or beverages.

Lifestyle changes

One change is focusing on consuming frequent, nutrient-dense meals and snacks, without consuming excessive calories during the pregnancy.

option for other family members.

wednesday	thursday	friday
iron-fortified cereal, wholewheat toast with margarine, kiwi fruit, skimmed milk	vegetable omelette, fresh fruit, wholewheat toast, skimmed milk	wholegrain scone with margarine, thick-cut bacon, fresh peach, skimmed milk
ham sandwich on wholegrain bread, chicken noodle soup, orange slices, skimmed milk	chicken salad sandwich on wholewheat bread, lentil soup, fresh strawberries, skimmed milk	vegetable wrap with provolone cheese, minestrone soup, mango slices, skimmed milk
lean steak, steamed cauliflower, baked sweet potato, watermelon, skimmed milk	baked pork loin, couscous, steamed fresh broccoli, fresh plum, skimmed milk	meatloaf, mashed potatoes, steamed carrots, fresh grapes, skimmed milk
bran muffin	apple slices with peanut butter	celery and carrot sticks with dip
low-fat yogurt drink	muesli bar	low-fat yogurt
pretzel sticks	fresh fruit	trail mix

Resources

www.womenshealth.gov/pregnancy

www.ific.org
(type "pregnancy" into search box)

Jones, C., Hudson, H. *Eating for Pregnancy* (2003, Marlowe and Company)

McHugh, M., Burggraf, E. *Your 9-Month Breakfast, Lunch, and Dinner Date* (2003, Eating for You (and Baby Too) Inc.)

LONG-TERM PLAN

FLEXIBILITY

FAMILY FRIENDLY

COST

STRENGTH OF SCIENCE

RAINBOW DIET

A plan that emphasizes eating colourful fresh fruit and vegetables for better health. Diet variations emphasize a spiritual connection between our bodies and how we nourish them.

How does it work?

The rationale behind the diet is that by eating a variety of foods of different colours, we are providing our bodies with vitamins and minerals. Vitamins, minerals, antioxidants and phytochemicals are attached to the pigments that colour fruit and vegetables. By making sure our plates are representative of the rainbow, we are likely to meet our daily food and nutrient requirements. This diet emphasizes high-fibre, low-calorie fruit and vegetables that are found to have disease-prevention and health-promoting properties. It has been well established by many research studies that eating five to nine servings of fruit and vegetables daily can help prevent some diseases.

Pros and cons

Following the plan helps ensure that the recommended servings of fruit and vegetables are included in the diet.

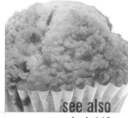

see also
dash 140
good mood 146
mypyramid 162

sample menu

This plan includes a variety of foods that

	saturday	sunday	monday	tuesday
morning	wholewheat toast, milk, grape juice, grapefruit	spinach and potato omelette, strawberries, milk	porridge, blueberries, milk, orange	tomato omelette, banana, wholewheat blueberry muffin
lunch	tuna salad on big mixed greens salad, tomatoes, asparagus, orange sherbet	vegetarian sub, kiwi fruit, low-sodium tomato juice, crisps	spinach salad, tomato slices, salmon, wholewheat bread	roast beef and Cheddar on rye, baked sweet potato fries, kiwi fruit
supper	minestrone soup, pasta primavera, baked pear with ginger glaze, red wine	paella with seafood and chicken, grilled plantains, okra with stewed tomatoes, olives, pomegranate	aubergine lasagne, carrots, mixed greens salad	white bean chilli, brown rice, spinach salad, courgettes
snack 1	dried mango and papaya chips	apples with cheese	yogurt, raspberries	yogurt, peach
snack 2	fruit salad	raw carrots and broccoli with dip	crackers with cheese	almonds

Eating a plateful of a large variety of colourful vegetables may promote a satiety (fullness from the fibre and water) and enhance weight loss.

The diet may provide plenty of information on consuming fruit and veggies, but it is limited in its advice on the other food groups. There are variations of this diet, which may recommend only organic foods or different amounts of foods from different groups, or only emphasize fruit and vegetables, so each diet must be carefully evaluated for nutritional adequacy and other claims.

healthy tips

- Beyond filling up on crunchy, sweet, tasty, and nourishing fruit and vegetables, plenty of water should be consumed.
- Choose heart-healthy nuts and lean meats, low-fat dairy and whole grains.
- Along with a plate of rainbow colours, choose foods that are low in saturated fats and high in fibre.

weigh this up...

What are phytochemicals? Phytochemicals are plant chemicals that have protective properties for health. The best way to make sure your diet includes phytochemicals is to eat them straight from the source – a variety of colourful fruit and vegetables. Eating natural, whole foods is always preferred over supplements. Among the most popular are lycopene in tomatoes, isoflavone in soya, and flavonoids found in red wine, dark chocolate and fruit.

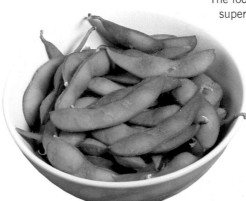

Is it for you?

This diet is likely to appeal to those who want to make their own food choices but need some direction or guidance. People who already possess some knowledge of nutrition, but need to include more high-fibre fruit and vegetables, will be interested in this diet.

People who have certain health conditions, such as diabetes, kidney or any other disease, should seek professional advice before starting this diet.

Availability

The foods can be found in most supermarkets.

Lifestyle changes

As part of overall health and well-being, a physical activity component is required.

emphasize freshness and colour.

wednesday	thursday	friday	Resources
peanut butter and banana sandwich, orange juice, skimmed milk	eggs, wholewheat toast, yogurt, strawberries	cereal with peach, skimmed milk	www.grinningplanet.com/2004/12-28/rainbow-diet-food-color-article.htm
vegetable soup, ½ turkey sandwich on wholewheat, blueberry parfait	carrots, green peas, collards, ham slices, corn bread, tomato salad	bean burrito, garden salad, vegetable juice, honeydew	
tofu and Chinese vegetable stir-fry with noodles, soya beans, cantaloupe	fish tacos with cilantro and fresh salsa, avocado, roasted root vegetables	lean sirloin, Brussels sprouts, winter squash, spinach and tomato salad	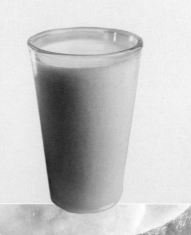
apple sauce	crackers with cheese and blackberries	three-berry smoothie with yogurt	
low-fat pudding	three-bean salad	red pepper strips	

LONG-TERM PLAN

FLEXIBILITY

FAMILY FRIENDLY

COST

STRENGTH OF SCIENCE

RAW FOOD DIET

This unconventional, radical eating guide consists of uncooked plant foods with "living enzymes".

Diet history

Raw foods were the first available natural biological food source. In the nineteenth century both Natural Hygiene Movement and a contemporary promoter called Herbert M. Shelton popularized the Raw Food Diet (of which there are many variations) in the United States. This eating strategy is moderately popular and typically used by vegetarians, celebrities and raw food restaurants.

How does it work?

The rationale for this radical lifestyle change advocates that foods in their raw state keep their health-promoting enzymes intact and their consumption results in major physiological shifts – improved energy levels, emotional balance, a delayed ageing process, a normalization in body weight, improved digestive processes, detoxification, a boosted immune system and lower triglyceride and cholesterol levels. Although grains, nuts, seeds and beans require soaking beforehand to activate the dormant enzymes, fruit and vegetables can be eaten without any preparation. Followers may include animal

wheatgrass

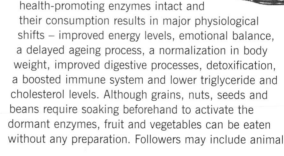

Bean and alfalfa sprouts are low in calories but may contain salmonella, so purchase them from a reliable source.

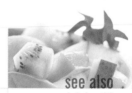

see also
juicing 90

sample menu

An increasing number of recipes for dishes made

	saturday	sunday	monday	tuesday
morning	raw prepared breakfast pizza	raw prepared bean salad	fruit, sprouts, seeds	fruit salad, avocado
lunch	fruit and vegetables with dip	coconut milk and fruit smoothie	wheatgrass, vegetable or fruit juice	fruit and vegetable
supper	gazpacho and crackers	lettuce wrap sandwich, sprout and veggie salad	raw prepared bread and sprout sandwich	raw prepared salad with soaked rice and beans

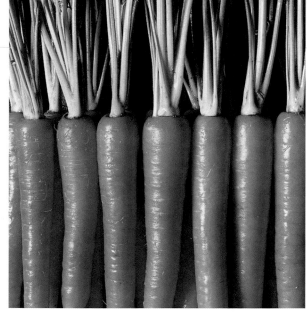

Carrots are an excellent source of beta carotene and a good source of fibre.

Is it for you?

This raw or a semi-raw plan may suit some vegetarians or naturalists who want to ingest food in an unprocessed state. Unfortunately, raw foods are the highest in pesticides so organic equivalents may be necessary which can be expensive. Individuals with compromised immune systems or digestive disorders, children, adolescents, and breastfeeding or pregnant women should not attempt it. A doctor and/or a registered dietician should be consulted beforehand.

Availability

All grocery shops or supermarkets will readily stock all the uncooked foods needed on this plan.

Lifestyle changes

The plan will require advanced menu planning, and shopping and preparation may take longer.

products or cooked foods in the diet but proponents claim the more raw the food, the better the health results.

The scientific evidence, however, suggests that some nutrients actually become more bio-available with cooking. The programme's elevated intake of fruit and vegetables has been associated with improved blood cholesterol and triglyceride levels.

Pros and cons

Raw food is easily digested and such a diet will refine digestion and increase the proportional intake of fruit and vegetables – also of fibre, water, some vitamins and minerals – while decreasing the calories and some fats. It is hard to overeat on the Raw Food Diet and easy to feel full without consuming many calories.

A diet consisting entirely of raw foods increases the risk of vitamin B12 deficiency so a supplement must be taken. Protein and calcium intake may also be low.

weigh this up...
- You can eat as little as 70% or as much as 100% raw food to become a true "raw foodist". Simply buy a food processor, juicer, blender and dehydrator – and you're all set to begin!

from raw foods are becoming available.

wednesday	thursday	friday
raw prepared cereal with nut milk	oatmeal chocolate smoothie	fruit, raw prepared cereal
fruit smoothie	fruit and vegetable with raw hummus	vegetable juice, sprouts
raw prepared sandwich with mushrooms	veggie salad with cheese and bread	raw prepared sandwich and fruit

Resources

www.living-foods.com

www.webmd.com/content

Rose, N. *Raw Food Life Force Energy* (2006, HarperCollins)

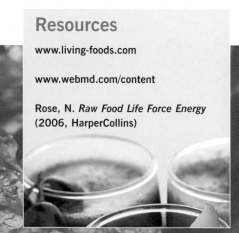

Note: There are many recipes for raw food cheeses, breads, pasta and soups.

LONG-TERM PLAN
●●●

FLEXIBILITY
●●●

FAMILY FRIENDLY
●●●

COST
●

STRENGTH OF SCIENCE
●●●

TLC DIET

Low in saturated fats, this programme reduces the likelihood of heart disease, heart attacks and other cardiovascular complications.

Diet history

The TLC (Therapeutic Lifestyle Change) Diet was adopted by the American Heart Association in 2001 based on guidelines for people with high cholesterol and risks of heart disease released by the NCEP (National Cholesterol Education Program) in its report.

How does it work?

The diet recommends that foods high in fibre and complex carbohydrates but low in unhealthy saturated fats and trans fats reduce cholesterol levels and avert the risk of heart disease. It advises obtaining between 25 per cent to 35 per cent or less of the day's total calories from fats, with less than 7 per cent of the total caloric intake from the unhealthy saturated variety and less than 200 milligrams of dietary cholesterol a day. Sodium allowance should also be limited and carbohydrates sourced mainly from whole grains, fruits and vegetables. Calories should be consumed to achieve or maintain a healthy stable

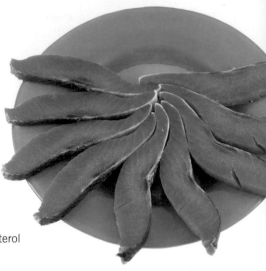
Fatty fish like salmon provides healthy Omega-3 fats to the diet.

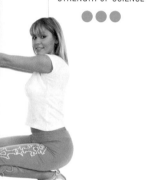

see also
mediterranean 160
omega 164

sample menu
The menu encourages healthy fats, whole grains,

	saturday	sunday	monday	tuesday
morning	French toast with 50g blueberries, soft margarine, maple syrup, orange, skimmed milk	smoothie (yogurt, 110g tofu, strawberries, blackberries) egg, 130g honeydew, 120ml skimmed milk	2-egg omelette with spinach and tomato, orange juice, skimmed milk	100g porridge with dried cherries, 120ml skimmed milk, orange juice
lunch	black bean soup with low-fat cheddar cheese, 100g brown rice, cantaloupe, unsweetened ice tea	baked halibut with couscous, summer squash, medium orange, skimmed milk	low-sodium turkey sandwich with sliced zucchini, small pouch-baked chips	corn tortilla with black beans and lean ground turkey, 2 tbsp salsa, unsweetened iced tea
supper	tuna fillet, green salad with vinaigrette, 2 small dinner rolls, skimmed milk	vegetable soup, veggie burger in bun, tomato salad, skimmed milk	grilled salmon, 100g couscous with pine nuts, 80g steamed broccoli, skimmed milk	wholeweat pasta baked with low-fat cheese and aubergine, small dinner roll, skimmed milk
snack 1	1 small corn tortilla, 100g refried beans	1 large banana	85g diced mango	1 small orange
snack 2	1 small peach	200g low-fat yogurt	2 tbsp prunes	65g walnuts

weight, and help reduce blood cholesterol levels. The scientific data to support these claims is strong.

Pros and cons

This AHA-endorsed diet is adequate in terms of vitamins, minerals, fibre, proteins, complex carbohydrates and healthy fat intake. Even though the plan is proven to help prevent cardiovascular disease, the assistance of a nutritional professional such as a registered dietician may be required to create a personalized food plan.

Is it for you?

The TLC Diet is likely to appeal to those who already suffer from or want to prevent heart disease, a heart attack or a stroke. Based on generic guidelines, the programme may also attract those who enjoy making their own food choices but may not be appropriate for individuals with certain medical conditions (such as kidney disease). Otherwise the diet is suitable for all, including those with diabetes and metabolic syndrome.

Availability

All the foods included in this diet are readily available and can be purchased from any general food shop.

Lifestyle changes

The diet suggests taking enough moderate exercise to expend at least 200 calories per day.

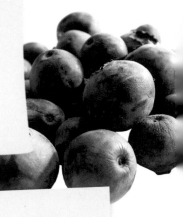

weigh this up...
- High-density lipoprotein (HDL) cholesterol is considered "good" cholesterol because it helps eliminate excess "bad" cholesterol from the body and protects the system.
- Low-density lipoprotein (LDL) is called "bad" cholesterol because it is deposited on the inside walls of the arteries once the body registers high levels.

healthy tips
- Ways of reducing high cholesterol include not smoking, losing and stabilizing weight and being physically active most days of the week.
- Bring blood cholesterol levels down by choosing foods low in saturated fats. Unhealthy fats raise the amounts of LDL or "bad" cholesterol and are found in fatty cuts of meats, poultry skin, whole dairy products, and tropical oils such as coconut and palm oils.

lean meats and low-fat dairy.

wednesday	thursday	friday	**Resources**
bran flakes, skimmed milk, orange, prune juice	1 muffin, 1 egg, 1 slice thick-cut bacon, unsweetened beverage	100g porridge with walnuts, skimmed milk, 1 small banana, toast, 1 tsp soft margarine	www.americanheart.org
salmon sandwich, tomato and cucumber salad, medium apple, skimmed milk	minestrone soup, 2 slices bread, 70g apple slices, skimmed milk	turkey sandwich with toast and light mayo, tomato juice	www.nhlbi.nih.gov/chd
roasted turkey, baked sweet potato, 80g Brussels sprouts, dinner roll, green salad, vinaigrette	linguine with prawns and low-sodium marinara sauce, watercress salad, chopped walnuts and vinaigrette, skimmed milk	grilled top-loin steak, 100g potatoes, 50g carrots, 2 small dinner rolls, skimmed milk	
200g low-fat yogurt	200g low-fat yogurt	1 low-fat cheese stick	
45g dried apricots	15g dry roasted almonds	75g carrot sticks	

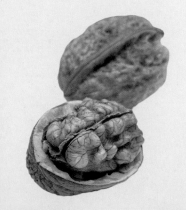

Note: All breads and buns are wholewheat.

LONG-TERM PLAN
●●●

FLEXIBILITY
●●●

FAMILY FRIENDLY
●●

COST
●●

STRENGTH OF SCIENCE
●●●

VEGAN DIET

Often referred to as "strict vegetarian", this eating plan excludes all fish, poultry, meat, eggs, dairy and any other animal by-products such as honey or animal gelatine.

Diet history

Coined in 1944 by Donald Watson, the word "vegan" was first published in *The Oxford Illustrated Dictionary* in 1962. The desire to separately identify dairy and non-dairy vegetarians prompted the beginnings of a coalition made up of non-dairy vegetarians. Donald Watson, Elsie Shrigley, and a few other like-minded individuals met in November 1944 in London to discuss the name of this new group. Although the term has not been around for that long, veganism has been practised for thousands of years. Although it is less commonly followed than some of the other vegetarian diets, the term is fairly well known.

How does it work?

Veganism is considered a lifestyle philosophy and not just a diet. Its rationale is based on ethical concerns for animal rights or the environment through the consumption of foods, thus eliminating animal products or by-products. Vegans also use plant-based products, and avoid leather, fur and any other items made from animal products including cosmetics and soaps.

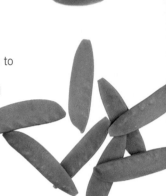

see also
lacto-ovo 150

sample menu
Product ingredients may vary, so always read the

	saturday	sunday	monday	tuesday
morning	cheese toast (wholewheat bread and vegan cheese), apple, grape juice	tofu scramblers, wholewheat toast with vegan margarine, kiwi, cranberry juice	wholewheat bagel, peanut butter, strawberries, orange juice	tofu scramblers, wholewheat toast, vegan margarine, banana, tea
lunch	soya hot dog on wholewheat bun, vegetarian baked beans, unsweetened applesauce, soya milk	veggie wholewheat crust pizza with vegan cheese, garden salad, oil and vinegar dressing, strawberries, soya milk	spinach salad with oranges, walnuts and raspberry vinaigrette, vegetable soup, wholewheat crackers, soya milk	tofu and veggie burrito, blue corn chips with salsa, pineapple, soya milk
dinner	green pepper stuffed with rice and tofu crumble, carrots, wholewheat dinner roll, pear, soya milk	tofu and veggie kebabs, couscous, mango, soya milk	grilled tempeh, broccoli with red peppers and onions, wild rice with pecans and raisins, plums, soya milk	nine-bean loaf, mashed cauliflower, green beans with flaked almonds, wheat dinner roll, vegan margarine, grapes, soya milk
snacks	wholewheat crackers with natural peanut butter, low-sodium vegetable juice with nutritional yeast	fruit smoothie (with soya, rice milk, yogurt or soft silken tofu), popcorn with nutritional yeast	low-sodium vegetable juice with nutritional yeast, cracker with nut butter	wholewheat pitta, hummus, nuts and dried fruit mix

Pros and cons
If nutritionally balanced, the Vegan Diet is a very healthy way of eating. Dining out, however, can be challenging and some vegan products are expensive.

Is it for you?
This diet is often followed for health or environmental reasons, out of concern for or in protest of the treatment of animals, or for religious reasons.

If planned carefully, the Vegan Diet is appropriate for anyone. You can eat as much of anything as you like that is allowed on the diet, but remember to choose foods and beverages 25 calories per serving or less to consume as "free" foods two to three times per day if you are limiting calories as well.

Since animal products contain vitamins B12 and D, it is important vegans obtain these and other vital nutrients (including calcium, iron, zinc and high-quality protein) from fortified, non-animal sources. Infants, children, teenagers, pregnant or breastfeeding women, or anyone new to the diet should have their eating habits examined by a dietician in advance to ensure nutritional adequacy.

Availability
Some vegan products can be expensive or hard to find.

Lifestyle changes
The Vegan Diet involves gradual behavioural adjustment in learning to identify items that contain animal substances or by-products.

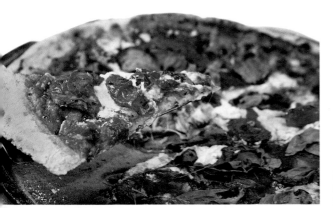

Veggie wholewheat crust pizza with vegan cheese.

healthy tips
- Look for products fortified with vitamins D and B12, calcium and iron.
- Complementary proteins do not have to be consumed in the same meal but need to be eaten within 24 hours.
- Use nutritional yeast to add vitamin B12 to your diet.
- Search for products with the vegan emblem when food shopping and use them to guide your selection.

label to ensure the product is vegan.

wednesday	thursday	friday
multigrain muffin, nut butter, cantaloupe and honeydew, apple juice	porridge, wholewheat muffin, vegan margarine, orange, tea	wholegrain cereal with soya milk, blueberries, orange juice
sandwich with veggie turkey slices, lettuce, tomato, tofu mayonnaise and alfalfa sprouts, lentil soup, fruit, soya milk	tofu reuben sandwich with vegan cheese, baked sweet potato chips, raspberries and blueberries, soya milk	vegetarian chilli (made with soya), peanut butter and jam sandwich on wholegrain bread, peaches, fortified soya milk
wholewheat pasta with marinara sauce, tofu crumbles and vegan parmesan, spinach, watermelon, soya milk	veggie burger on wholegrain bun with lettuce, tomato, onion, tofu mayonnaise and vegan cheese, roasted red potatoes with olive oil, fruit kebab, soya milk	aubergine parmesan made with vegan cheese, asparagus, wholewheat dinner roll, vegan margarine, apricots, soya milk
fruit, popcorn with nutritional yeast	celery sticks, hummus, vegan ice cream topped with wheatgerm	wholegrain bagel, nut butter, soya yogurt with fruit

Resources
www.vrg.org

www.americanvegan.org

www.veganviews.org.uk/vvcrossref.html

Stepaniak, J., Messina, V., Adams, C.J. *The Vegan Sourcebook* (2000, McGraw Hill)

Wasserman, D., Mangels, R. *Simply Vegan* (2006, Vegetarian Resource Group)

Note: Soya or rice milk and juices should be fortified with calcium, vitamin D and vitamin B12. Look for the vegan emblem on food products.

WHAT WOULD JESUS EAT?

Described as "the ultimate programme for eating well, feeling great and living longer", this diet is based on foods similar to those that Jesus may have consumed.

LONG-TERM PLAN

FLEXIBILITY

FAMILY FRIENDLY

COST

STRENGTH OF SCIENCE

Diet history
Dr Colbert, a physician, is the author of this book and corresponding programme. Throughout the book, Dr Colbert quotes and interprets Biblical scriptures, from which he extrapolates and lists foods and beverages that Jesus would have consumed during his life.

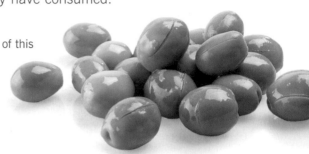

How does it work?
The diet encourages healthy eating. Foods that, according to Dr Colbert, Jesus would have consumed are encouraged and other foods are discouraged. Dr Colbert purports that Jesus consumed many fruits, vegetables, kosher meats and whole grains, and did not consume animal fats. Thus, in this meal plan, olive oil is the main fat source; "butter" in Jesus' time was mainly olive oil. Also, fish, not other meat, was more popular in Jesus' day. It is thought that he ate fish and bread almost daily. According to Dr Colbert, manna, or bread from heaven, was thought to be bread during the time of Jesus.

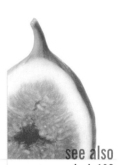

see also
dash 138
mediterranean 160

sample menu
This plan assumes that Jesus primarily ate fruits,

	saturday	sunday	monday	tuesday
morning	120ml freshly squeezed orange juice, omelette with vegetables, wholegrain toast	oat bran cereal with sliced almonds, small orange, 120ml water	120ml freshly squeezed, orange juice, porridge with walnuts and blackberries	wholegrain cereal with fresh strawberries and skimmed milk, 110ml water
lunch	vegetable soup, wholegrain bread, dark green salad with walnuts, water	black bean soup, wholegrain pitta with hummus, water	Greek salad with feta cheese, wholewheat pitta with hummus, water	tuna salad (water-packed) on cos lettuce, wholegrain bread, water
supper	wholegrain penne pasta with marinara sauce, steamed broccoli with Parmesan cheese, 120ml water	grilled white fish, brown rice, steamed courgettes, wholewheat bread, 120ml red wine	grilled salmon, spinach salad, wholewheat bread, steamed asparagus, 120ml red wine	baked sea bass, steamed green beans, wild rice, lentil soup, 120ml water
snack 1	fresh pear and water	fresh mango slices and water	blueberries with low-fat plain yogurt	cantaloupe with fat-free cottage cheese
snack 2	grapefruit	fresh pineapple, fat-free or low-fat cottage cheese	water and small apple	kiwi and water

This meal plan is rich in fresh fruit and vegetables, different types of fish, whole grains, olive oil, lentils and chickpeas. Stevia, a sweet herb, is recommended instead of using sugar or artificial sweeteners. Consuming small portions and fruit for dessert are encouraged. Over-consumption of high-calorie and high-fat foods is discouraged, especially foods rich in saturated fat. Eliminating processed foods is encouraged. The science data support that a diet high in fruit, vegetables, whole grains, fish and olive oil is health promoting.

Pros and cons

Drinking water is encouraged. Healthy, nutrient-rich foods are promoted. Simple and healthy recipes are provided. There is also a separate cookery book available.

The disadvantage is that completely avoiding processed foods may be unrealistic and discouraging for some.

Although the book does not recommend supplements they are sold/promoted on the website which seems contradictory to the diet.

Is it for you?

This meal plan is designed for individuals who are interested in eating the way it is thought that Jesus ate, based on the Biblical scriptures, on the assumption that it is health promoting. Individuals trying to lose weight may also be interested in this meal plan.

The foods in this meal plan are healthy and are appropriate for nearly everyone. However, calories and portion sizes of the foods should be tailored to meet individual calorie and nutrient needs. This is especially important for children, adolescents, and pregnant or breastfeeding women. The red wine should be excluded for these individuals as well.

Availability

Most foods are easily accessible and available. There are some speciality foods and drinks, and a few items may be unfamiliar (for example stevia – a natural herb sweetener) and slightly more difficult to find.

Lifestyle changes

Food behaviour changes, such as always eating breakfast, making lunch the main meal, eating an early and light dinner, and choosing fruit for desserts and snacks are encouraged. Increasing physical activity is also emphasized.

healthy tips
- Choose skimmed-milk products or 1%-fat dairy products.
- Eat slowly.
- Eat more fresh fruit and vegetables.
- Avoid fried foods.

vegetables, whole grains and kosher meats.

wednesday	thursday	friday
120ml freshly squeezed orange juice, wholegrain toast, soya sausage, grapefruit	120ml freshly-squeezed grapefruit juice, high-fibre cereal with raspberries and skimmed milk	plain fat-free yogurt with fresh blueberries, small apple, wholegrain toast, 120ml water
grilled chicken breast sandwich on wholegrain bread, steamed broccoli with red pepper, water	lentil soup, wholegrain pitta with hummus, water	spinach salad with feta cheese and olive oil and vinegar dressing, wholegrain bread, water
thin-crusted wholewheat vegetable pizza, garden salad, 120ml red wine	grilled white fish, steamed cauliflower and carrots, wholegrain bread, 120ml water	baked chicken breast, steamed snap peas, wholegrain couscous, 120ml red wine
watermelon and water	plum and water	grapes and water
fat-free or low-fat plain yogurt with fruit	fresh melon, fat-free or low-fat cottage cheese	raspberries and fat-free or low-fat plain yogurt

Resources

www.DrColbert.com

Colbert, D. *What Would Jesus Eat? The Ultimate Program for Eating Well, Feeling Great, and Living Longer* (2002, Thomas Nelson)

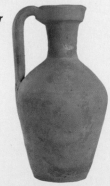

Notes: Water should be bottled or filtered, with lemon or lime juice and stevia added if desired. Bread and toast can have extra virgin olive oil with them. Salads include a vinegar and olive oil dressing.

GLOSSARY

Alcohol
Also known as ethanol, alcohol is a depressant made from fermented sugars. It provides 7 calories per gram.

Calorie dense
Foods that are high in calories and usually low in nutrients. Also referred to as empty-calorie foods. (See nutrient dense.)

Carbohydrate
Compounds made of single (simple) or multiple (complex) sugars. Meaning "carbon and water", they play an important role in body metabolism and immunity. Recommended daily intake is usually between 50–75 per cent of total calories, with less than 10 per cent coming from simple sugars based on adequate caloric intake for healthy weight maintenance.

Cortisol
A hormone released during times of stress. It raises blood pressure and blood sugar levels, and may suppress the immune system.

Energy
The capacity to do work. Energy from food is measured in, and referred to as, calories and is absorbed during digestion.

Fats
Consist of a large group of compounds, known as lipids that are either solid (fats) or liquid (oils) at room temperature. Fats play a role in body temperature regulation, cell function and organ insulation. Eating too much of the solid fats can lead to cardiovascular disease, while eating liquid oils have protective qualities. Recommended intake is approximately 30 per cent of total calories based on adequate caloric intake for healthy weight maintenance.

Fibre, dietary
The non-starchy parts of plant foods that are not digested. Rather, they move through the digestive system, absorbing water and cholesterol. There are two types of dietary fibre: soluble and non-soluble. Soluble fibre dissolves in water; non-soluble does not.

Food exchange system
A diet-planning tool that groups foods according to their nutrient content and/or calories. The diabetes food exchange system ensures that the same calories or grams of carbohydrates are being consumed. There are many varieties of food exchange systems. The systems are beneficial in planning a varied diet that includes different types of foods.

Glucose
A carbohydrate that is a simple sugar. It is the body's main source of energy and is used in metabolism. It is essential, and the only form of energy used by the nervous system and red blood cells.

Glycogen
Glucose stored in the liver and muscles, used when blood glucose levels are low.

Grazing
Eating several (five or more) small meals a day versus three large meals.

HDL
A high-density lipoprotein. Considered the "good cholesterol", levels of about at least 1 mmol/litre or higher have been shown to be protective against heart disease.

Ketosis
A stage in metabolism when glucose is not present. During ketosis, fat is converted into ketone bodies to be used for metabolism.

Lactose
The sugar in milk. It is digested with the help of the enzyme lactase, which breaks down lactose into two simple sugars called glucose and galactose. If the person does not produce enough or any lactose, he or she may have difficulty digesting unfermented milk products. Among the symptoms are bloating and gas, and mild to severe nausea, cramps, and diarrhoea. Symptom severity depends on the amount

of lactose tolerated, digestion rate, meal combination, etc. This lactose intolerance is sometimes confused with milk allergy, which is an immune-system reaction to the proteins, not the sugars, in milk.

Leptin
A hormone that plays a role in regulating appetite and metabolism.

LDL
A low-density lipoprotein. Considered the "bad cholesterol", levels of above 4 mmol/litre have been shown to be a major risk factor in heart disease.

Medical nutrition therapy
MNT, as it is known, is commonly defined as "nutritional diagnostic, therapeutic, and counselling services for the purpose of disease management which are furnished by a registered dietician or nutrition professional". It was previously known as diet therapy.

Metabolic syndrome
A combination of insulin resistance or high fasting blood sugar, central obesity, hypertension, low HDL-cholesterol, and high blood triglycerides that increases a person's risk of cardiovascular disease.

Mineral
Inorganic non-calorie (energy) elements found in varying degrees in human bodies and in the earth. Each required mineral plays a specific role in the body. In nutrition, the major minerals include calcium, phosphorus, sodium, potassium, magnesium, chloride and sulphate.

Monounsaturated fats
Derive their name from the chemical structure, which has one fatty acid with one point of unsaturation. These fats are liquid at room temperature and are mostly found in plant (vegetable) oils such as olive oil. This type of fat may help raise HDL cholesterol.

Nutrient dense
A nutrient-dense food is high in a nutrient relative to calories; that is, the ratio of nutrient content (in grams) to the total energy (calorie) content is high. For example, skimmed milk is nutrient dense with calcium. Nutrient-dense foods provide a large amount of vitamins and minerals with few calories, for example, fruits and vegetables. (See calorie dense.)

Nutrigenomics
The integration of the genetics and other sciences to human nutrition. This is a new discipline that is expected to affect future nutrition care because differences in genotype should impact on the relationship between diet and health at individual levels.

Omega-3 and Omega-6 fats
These polyunsaturated fats have varying functions in the human body. Soya, sunflower and some other vegetable oils are good sources of Omega-6 fats. Seafood, especially fatty fish, is a good source of Omega-3 fats, which are reported to provide heart healthy benefits.

Phytochemicals
Compounds or chemicals found in plants that are not required but have been found to be beneficial to health. Also called phytonutrients.

Polyunsaturated fats
Derive their name from the chemical structure, which has fatty acids with more than one point of unsaturation. These fats are liquid in room temperature and may help reduce total cholesterol.

Portion control
Knowing and understanding what a serving size is for a food and how many calories a serving contains. Typical serving sizes have ballooned into bigger sizes, which may have contributed to expanding waistlines.

Protein
Compounds made up of multiple arrangements of amino acids, some of which are not made by the body and must therefore be obtained through foods (essential amino acids). Proteins are found in cells, enzymes, muscles, and other structures in the human body. Protein intake should be within 10–35 per cent of total adequate calories.

Sparing of body protein
The process by which the energy provided by carbohydrates and fats allows protein to be used for functions it alone can provide.

Structured eating
A diet or menu plan with a routine meal pattern, or that has specific rules or guidelines that may be restrictive and designed to be regular in timing. For example, eating three meals a day with an evening snack.

Thermic effect
The amount of energy (calories) that the body uses to metabolize the food consumed.

Trans fats
Mostly occur as a result of creating a solid fat from a liquid oil through the process of partial hydrogenation of plant oils. However, trans fats also occur in small quantities in some meat and dairy products. Trans fats are not required in the diet and have been associated with increased risk of heart disease.

Vitamins
Non-caloric compounds of nutrients that are required in very small amounts and are essential for metabolism. Deficiency of these compounds may be harmful. Vitamins are divided into two groups: fat soluble and water soluble. Fat-soluble vitamins include A, D, E, and K. Water-soluble vitamins include B and C.

BIBLIOGRAPHY

Airola, P. *How to Keep Slim, Healthy, and Young with Juice Fasting* (1971, Health Plus Publ.)

Adamson, E., Horning, L. *The Complete Idiot's Guide to Fasting* (2002, Alpha Books)

Agatston, A. *The South Beach Diet* (2003, St. Martin's Press)

American Dietetic Association *ADA Nutrition Care Manual* (2007, American Dietetic Association)

Atkins, R. *Dr. Atkin's New Diet Revolution* (2002, HarperCollins)

Audette, R. *Neanderthin* (1999, St. Martin's Press)

Beale, L., Couvillon, S.G., Clark, J. *The Complete Idiot's Guide to Healthy Weight Loss* (2005, Alpha)

Brand-Miller, J., Foster-Powell, K., McMillan-Price, J. *The Low GI Diet Revolution* (2004, Marlowe and Co.)

Burrell, D. *Psychology Today: Secrets of Successful Weight Loss* (2006, Alpha Books)

Burroughs, S. *The Master Cleanser* (1976, Burroughs Books; Revised Ed., Burroughs, A. 1993)

Case, S. *Gluten-Free Diet – A Comprehensive Resource Guide* (2006, Case Nutrition Consulting)

Cloutier, M., Adamson, E. *The Mediterranean Diet* (2004, HarperCollins)

Colbert, D. *What Would Jesus Eat? The Ultimate Program for Eating Well, Feeling Great, and Living Longer* (2002, Thomas Nelson)

Conley, R. *The Complete Hip and Thigh Diet* (1989, Warner Books, Inc.)

Connolly Schoonen, J. *Losing Weight Permanently with the Bull's-Eye Food Guide* (2004, Bull Publishing Company)

Craig, J. *The Jenny Craig Story: How One Woman Changes Millions of Lives* (2004, John Wiley & Sons, Inc.)

Crook, W. G. *The Yeast Connection and Women* (1998, Professional Books)

Cruise, J. *The 3-Hour Diet* (2006, HarperCollins)

D'Adamo, P., Whitney, C. *Eat Right For Your Type* (1996, GP Putnam & Sons)

Danbrot, M. *The New Cabbage Soup Diet* (2004, St. Martin's Press)

Diamond, H., Diamond, M. *Fit for Life* (1985, Warner Books)

Duyff, R. (American Dietetic Association Staff) *American Dietetic Association Complete Food and Nutrition Guide* (2006, Wiley, John & Sons)

Elisabeth, L. *Twelve Steps for Overeaters* (1993, Hazelden Publications)

Feingold, B. & Feingold, H. *The Feingold Cookbook for Hyperactive Children* (1979, Random House)

Florida Dietetic Association *Florida Manual of Medical Nutrition Therapy* (2007)

Flynn, T. *The 3-Apple-a-Day Plan* (2005, Broadway Books)

Fox, M., Burros, L. *Pure and Simple: Delicious Recipes for Additive-Free Cooking* (1978, Berkley Publishing Group)

Gallop, R. *Living the GI Diet* (2004, Workman Publishing Co.)

Glickman, P. *Lose Weight, Have More Energy & Be Happier in 10 Days* (2005, Glickman, Peter, Inc.)

Green, B. *The Best Life Diet* (2006, Simon & Schuster)

Guiliano, M. *French Women Don't Get Fat: The Secret of Eating for Pleasure* (2005, Random House)

Gutterson, C. *The Sonoma Diet* (2005, Meredith Books)

Hastings, J. *Change One* (2003, Reader's Digest)

Heber, D. *The New LA Shape Diet: The 14-Day Total Weight Loss Plan* (2004, Regan Books)

Hirsch, A. R. *Scentsational Weight Loss: At Last a New Easy Natural Way To Control Your Appetite* (1997, Element Books, Inc.)

Howard, A., Marks, J. *The Cambridge Diet: A Manual for Practitioners* (1986, MTP Press)

Huerta S, Li z, Li MS, et al. *Feasibility of a partial meal replacement plan for weight loss in low income patients* Internat. J Obesity (2004) 28;1575

Hutton, L., Kotz, D. *The Slim-Fast Body, Mind, Life Makeover* (2000, HarperCollins)

Hyman, M. *The UltraSimple Diet* (2007, Pocket Books, Simon & Schuster)

Hyman, M. *UltraMetabolism* (2006, Simon & Schuster)

Jameson, G., Williams, E. *The Drinking Man's Diet, revised edition* (2004, Cameron & Co.)

Jibrin, J. *Good Housekeeping Book: The Supermarket Diet* (2007, Hearst, Sterling Publishing Co., Inc.)

Jones, C., Hudson, H. *Eating for Pregnancy* (2003, Marlowe and Company)

Katahn, M. *The Tri-Color Diet* (1996, W. W. Norton & Co.)

Katzen, M., Willett, W. *Eat, Drink, and Weigh Less* (2006, Hyperion)

Kirby, J. (American Dietetic Association Staff) *Dieting For Dummies* (2003, Wiley, John & Sons)

Kirsch, D. *The Ultimate New York Diet* (2006, McGraw Hill)

Kleiner, S. *The Good Mood Diet* (2005, Springboard Press)

Kushi, M., Jack, A. *The Macrobiotic Path to Total Health* (2003, Ballantine Books)

Magee, E. *Tell Me What to Eat If I Have Acid Reflux: Nutrition You Can Live With* (2002, The Career Press)

Marsden, K. *The Food Combining Diet: Lose Weight the Hay Way* (1993, Thorsons)

Mazel, J., Wyatt, M. *The New Beverly Hills Diet* (1996, Health Communications, Inc.)

McCord, H. *The Peanut Butter Diet* (2001, St. Martin's Paperbacks)

McHugh, M., Burggraf, E. *Your 9-Month Breakfast, Lunch, and Dinner Date* (2003, Eating for You (and baby too), Inc.)

Messina, V., Messina, M. *The Vegetarian Way* (1996, Three Rivers Press)

Mitchell, S., Christie, C. *Fat is Not Your Fate: Outsmart Your Genes and Lose Weight Forever* (2006, Simon & Schuster, Inc.)

Mitchell, S., Christie, C. *I'd Kill For a Cookie* (1998, Plume)

Noakes M., Foster P.R., Koegh J.B., Clifton P.M. *Meal Replacement as effective as structured weight loss diets for treating obesity in adults with features of metabolic syndrome* J Nutr. (2004) 134;8

Ornish, D. *Eat More, Weigh Less* (2002, Quill, HarperCollins)

Overeaters Anonymous (2001, Overeaters Anonymous Inc.)

Perricone, N. *The Perricone Promise* (2004, Warner Books)

Principal, V. *Living Principal* (2001, Villard)

Principal, V. *The Diet Principal* (1987, Simon & Schuster)

Pritikin, R. *The New Pritikin Program* (1991, Simon & Schuster)

Pritikin, R. *The Pritikin Principle* (2000, Time Life)

Purcella, G., Cabot, S., Barry-Dee, C. *Juice Fasting Bible* (2007, Ulysses Press)

Rinzler, C., Kristal, L. *Nutrition For Dummies* (2006, Wiley, John & Sons)

Rodriguez, J. *Contemporary Nutrition for Latinos* (2004, iUniverse)

Roizen, M.F., Oz, M.C. *You, On a Diet* (2005, Simon & Schuster)

Rolls, B. *The Volumetrics Eating Plan* (2007, HarperCollins)

Rolls, B., Barnett, R. *The Volumetrics Weight-Control Plan* (2002, Harper)

Rose, N. *Raw Food Life Force Energy* (2006, HarperCollins)

Rose W. C. *The amino acid requirements of adult man* Nutr. Abst. Rev., (1957) 27;631

Rosedale, R., Colman, C. *The Rosedale Diet* (2004, Harper Resource)

Rouse, J. *NutriSystem Nourish: The Revolutionary New Weight Loss Program* (2004, John Wiley & Sons, Inc.)

Scales, MJ. *Diets in a Nutshell* (2006, Apex Publishers)

Sears, B. *The Zone* (1995, HarperCollins)

Simopoulos, A.P., Robinson, J. *The Omega Plan* (1998, HarperCollins)

Sizer, F., Whitney, E. *Nutrition Concepts and Controversies* (2006, Brooks/Cole)

Somers, S. *Get Skinny on Fabulous Food* (1999, Crown Publications)

Somers, S. *Suzanne Somers' Fast and Easy* (2002, Crown Publications)

Stepaniak, J., Messina, V., Adams, C.J. *The Vegan Sourcebook* (2000, McGraw Hill Co.)

Steward, H. L., Bethea, M., Andrews, S., Balart, L. *The New Sugar Busters! Cut Sugar To Trim Fat* (2003, Ballantine Books)

Tarnower, H., Sinclair-Baker, S. *The Complete Scarsdale Medical Diet Plus Dr. Tarnower's Lifetime Keep-Slim Program* (1978, Bantam Books)

The Mayo Clinic Plan 10 Essential Steps to a Better Body and Healthier Life (2006, Time, Inc.)

Thompson, DL., Ahrens, MJ. *The Grapefruit Solution* (2004, Linx Corp.)

Thompson, J., Manore, M. *Nutrition: An Applied Approach* (2005, Pearson Education)

Tribole, E., Resch, E. *Intuitive Eating* (2003, 2nd ed., St. Martin's Press)

Turby H., Baic S., deLooy A. et al. *Randomized controlled trial of four commercial weight loss programs from BBC "diet trials"* Bristish Medical Journal doi:10.1136/bmj.38833.411204.80 (2006)

US Department of Health and Human Services *Your guide to lowering your blood pressure with the DASH* (2006, National Institute of Health, National Heart, Lung, and Blood Institute, NIH Pub 06-4082)

Wasserman, D., Mangels, R. *Simply Vegan* (2006, Vegetarian Resource Group)

Woloshyn, T. *Complete Master Cleanse: A Step by Step Guide to Maximizing the Benefits of the Lemonade Diet* (2007, Ulysses Press)

Woodruff, S. *Secrets of Good-Carb Low-Carb Living* (2004, Avery)

Zinczenko, D. *The Abs Diet* (2004, Rodale, Inc.)

INDEX

CREDITS

I would like to thank my husband, George, and family for their never-ending support of my personal and professional endeavours. Many thanks also to the Nutrition faculty who helped write the book, to Dr Jacquie Fraser and UNF students who helped with the research, and to the University of North Florida, for providing the time and resources necessary to work on the book.

Quarto would also like to acknowledge the following:

p12
United States Department of Health & Human Services
www.dhhs.gov
200 Independence Avenue, S.W.
Washington, D.C. 20201
Tel: 202-619-0257 Toll Free: 1-877-696-6775

Quarto would like to acknowledge the following photographers from ©iStockphoto.com for the use of their pictures reproduced in this book:

Key: a = above, b = below, c = centre, l = left, r = right

Monika Adamczyk	120r
Roberto Adrian	136–137b, 174–175b
Chris Bence	156–157b
Arpad Benedek	166–167a
William Berry	162r
Michael Blackburn	46r
Jennifer Borton	40–41a
Trevor Buttery	67a
Joanne C.W. Chang	66–67b
Libby Chapman	154r
Kelly Cline	42r, 64r, 86–87b, 92r, 110–111b, 152–153b
Creacart	32r
Pablo Eder	40–41b
Liv Friis-Larsen	46–47b, 90–91b, 106–107b, 174r, 175b
Peter Garbet	156–157a
Daniel Gilbey	106c
Smantha Grandy	46–47a
David Hernandez	113r
Momchil Hristov	106a
Paul Johnson	33c

kkgas	179c
Satu Knape	154–155b
Olaf Kowalzik	110b
Anthony Ladd	111b
Guillermo Lobo	41cr
Jason Lugo	49a
Olga Lyubkina	53r, 90r (red)
Alexander Maksimenko	88r
Carmen MartÃnez BanÃs	70–71a
James McQuillan	91r, 120–121a
Prill Mediendesign & Fotografie	102–103a
Anna Milkova	59a
Juan Monino	58r
Sang Nguyen	156r
Christine Nichols	67b
Chepe Nicoli	93l
pdcamp	87b
Kristian Peetz	33r, 86l
Marcel Pelletier	64–65b
Ina Peters	28r, 86–87a
Paul Reid	93br
Amanda Rohde	86r
Sasimoto	155l
Nina Shannon	90r (purple)
Olga Shelego	112r
Roman Sigaev	70r
Suzannah Skelton	40r, 52r
Liz van Steenburgh	29b
Jason Stitt	65a, 93r
Mark Stout	174l
Suprijono Suharjoto	43r, 44b
Denise Torres	174–175a
Joan Vicent Cantó Roig	161r
Graça Victoria	41cl
Craig Veltri	92–93a

All other pictures are the copyright of Quarto Publishing plc. Whilst every effort has been made to credit contributors, Quarto would like to apologize should there have been any omissions or errors – and would be pleased to make the appropriate correction for future editions of the book.